Supermen

Building Maximum Muscle for a Lifetime

Craig Cecil

Supermen: Building Maximum Muscle for a Lifetime

Copyright © 2011 by Craig Cecil.

ISBN: 978-0-9847414-1-0
ISBN: 978-0-9847414-0-3 (ebook)

First edition: November 2011

Manufactured in the United States of America

Trademarked names may appear in this book. Rather than use a trademark symbol with every occurrence of a trademarked name, we use the names only in an editorial fashion and to the benefit of the trademark owner, with no intention of infringement of the trademark.

Warning: Before beginning any exercise program, consult with your physician to ensure that you are in proper health. This book does not provide medical or therapeutic advice; you should obtain medical advice from your healthcare practitioner. Before starting any new program, check with your doctor, especially if you have a specific physical problem or are taking any medication. No liability is assumed by the author or publisher for any of the information contained herein.

Disclaimer: Steroids, HGH, Diuretics and any other Illegal Performance Enhancing Drugs

Illegal substances are endemic in our society. They have permeated all aspects of modern culture—sports, entertainment, and high school and middle school age children. They have no place in this book or the concepts presented herein.

The true measure of a person is not the muscle they carry or the physical strength they possess, but the character within. Be true to yourself and others.

Cover design: Jaclyn Urlahs

Contents

Weak Point Training 135

How to Work Out When You Are Injured........................ 141

Thanks!

This book is dedicated to all those who have gone on the journey with me, including mentors, friends, willing participants, unwitting suspects, innocent bystanders, and past and future champions.

Thanks to Mitch, Nathan, Mad Dog, Jason, Dave, Willie, Mark, Rob, Adam, and Kyle. Whether you realized it or not, you helped validate the system and concepts in this book.

I probably couldn't have done it without you—nah, yes I could ☺

Mitch, you deserve a medal for training with me for over two decades. I hope I've helped keep you young and you've helped keep me grounded (there's still hope!). No one could ask for a better friend—how I deserved you, only God knows.

Oh, and a very special thanks to Leslie, who put up with it all. Still.

Tell Me What You Think

I'm always interested in getting feedback on my books. Please send your comments and suggestions to:

books@runningdeersoftware.com

Introduction

This book presents a weightlifting system that maximizes the muscular development of an individual, while creating a complete, balanced and symmetrical physique. It is not a guide for maximizing strength, increasing your bench press, or cutting up for a physique contest. It's not a manual for how to perform basic weightlifting movements. It's a book that will save you years of trial-and-error in the gym and provide you with decades of weight training insights. It's a book for the rest of us—those with average genetics, strong minds and stronger hearts. More significantly, it represents a long-term plan for lifting weights wisely throughout your life while building and maintaining significant muscle mass.

The application of consistent, logical effort, over a prolonged period is the key to reaching your physical muscular potential. For most individuals, that means training smart and training hard for at least three years. In that time, an ordinary individual can transform into a virtual superman among his peers.

This book will show you how to do it.

Origins

It all started in the summer of 1989.

I had just finished my undergraduate degree and was preparing to go off to graduate school. My NCAA Track & Field career had just ended. Before that, I had made the move from baseball (Little League through high school ball). I had always been active, always played sports. Now, I was at a crossroads.

What do I do now? I knew I wanted to pick something that I could do for the rest of my life. I ran through the usual suspects in my head—golf (too time consuming, frustrating, weather dependent), bowling (not active enough), billiards, darts, ping-pong (you're kidding, right?).

Then, I remembered my uncle. He came by to visit every so often and man, did he have some guns on him. In fact, he was heavily muscled, especially for a man who stood about five foot seven—and, he had managed to win a state bodybuilding contest while training at home. His son had accomplished similar feats and was still going strong in the competitive amateur bodybuilding world. I wondered if there might be some genetic potential…

During college, I was supposed to do some off-season conditioning in the weight room in preparation for track and field season. I don't think I even touched any free weights, just air-pressurized Keiser machines. (The college installed those machines exclaiming that they were greater than sliced bread—guess which was always broken, the machines or the cast iron free weights?) I trudged into the weight room about two or three times a week (more often two) for a few weeks before track season every year. Didn't see any difference—no big surprise there.

Four years later, I saw the same image staring back at me in the mirror that I saw as a freshman—5'11" and 165 lbs with some (very) minor muscle separation. Probably 14% body fat. It was time to do something about this. My initial goal was to try to put on about 20 lbs of muscle, taking me up to 185 lbs. At my height, I thought that would give me a nice, slightly muscular look. I might even turn the heads of some ladies. Isn't that why most of us guys lift weights anyway?

Now, you have to understand that when I decide to jump into something, it's all or nothing. There is no middle ground. With that in mind, in very short order I bought Arnold's *Encyclopedia of Modern Bodybuilding*, altered my diet to include a LOT more protein and calories, bought a simple weight set and bench, then joined a gym and started working out 5-6 days per week. Hard.

I mean really hard.

Every set to failure hard.

Very quickly, I noticed that I was making rapid progress. I also noted that I was doing two things that most others in the gym were not doing—I was feeding my body a truckload of protein and calories, and I was working out very, very hard *consistently*.

Fast forward ten years and the image in the mirror staring back was vastly different; in fact, the transformation was nothing short of amazing—5'11" and 260 lbs with 10% body fat. I had created a virtual superman. Except this one was real.

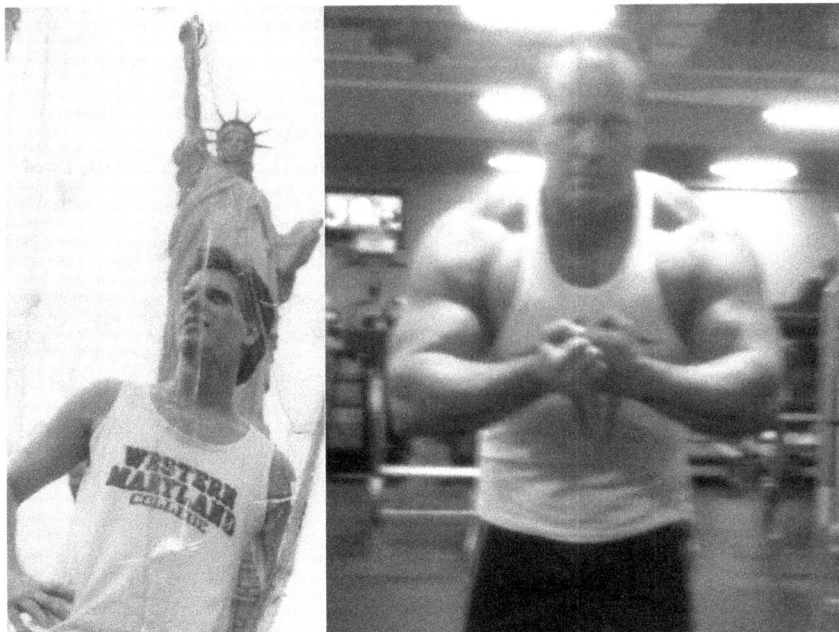

(Sorry about the quality of the photos above, but I wanted you to see un-retouched, raw photos. The before picture of me was taken a couple weeks before I started lifting weights—this is what I looked like through high school and college. The after picture was taken with an iPhone right before publication of this book. I used no performance enhancing drugs—ever. Oh, and I only worked biceps before the picture was taken—everything else is un-pumped.)

The system worked—for me. But did it work for others as well?

Over the past twenty years, I've been fortunate to have a small army of dedicated training partners follow my steps. One has been with me for the entire twenty-plus year saga, several others have been around for more than a decade, and the rest of the current cadre have endured a solid five-year tenure. Even more have come in and out of the training circle for periods of 3 months to a year. In all, about one hundred trained under my system for at least three solid months over the last twenty years.

Some came with years of weight training experience, others with a couple years, and still others were practically new to weights. Some were tall, others short, some naturally muscular, others lean, overweight, or skinny.

For those who followed my system for at least three months, one thing was always constant—they ended up at their leanest, most muscular body weight they ever achieved. Over those 20 years, I built an army of supermen.

So in the end, my system worked for all who followed it as prescribed, I got the girl (she's now my wife), and I learned a lot of valuable lessons which I've tried to capture in this book.

Now, let's start your transformation and get to the good stuff.

Guiding Principles

The system presented in this book has the same guiding principles as almost every other weightlifting system created. Except, we're going to add one more that most don't talk about—intelligence. You'll see how it makes a big difference. Along the way, we'll also ask for courage, honesty, and a little critical thinking. They all add up to success.

● Consistency

Showing up really is half the battle. The thing is, you've got to show up all the time, week after week, month after month, year after year. This is not a sprint—it's a marathon. It ends when you end. There's a reason that grueling long-term events are called 'Iron Man' events. In this case, you're going to build Iron Man. Remember, it's all about building momentum. There can be no periods of starting and stopping. You need to work out consistently. It's you versus you. The most important principle. End of discussion.

● Progressive Resistance

Now that you're showing up all the time, you need to continually do things that increase the stress on your muscles (if you don't, nothing is going to change). This is called progressive resistance—it's the bedrock of all weightlifting systems. In this book, you'll become a magician at combining the elements of weight, time and volume to produce exceptional results. Doing exceptional things will produce exceptional results. I'll give you plenty of exceptional workouts in the second half of this book that are guaranteed to increase the stress on your muscles.

● Compound, Multi-Joint Movements with Full Range of Motion

You show up all the time, you're a master of progressive resistance training, but you still aren't growing muscles like you want. Stop using the cable-crossover and start basing the core of every workout around compound, multi-joint movements. You know them. They're the ones that everyone likes to avoid: squats, front-squats, deadlifts, cleans, rows, and chins. Get past the bench press and there's a world of these exercises. I'll show you how to combine them effectively with isolation exercises to create that superhero physique you really want. It's simple. Don't include basic, compound movements as the core of every workout and don't get a supremely muscular physique. I'll talk more about this below.

Additionally, you need to use a full range of motion with all exercises in order to build a complete physique. Half-reps may build your ego but they also build half a physique. There is a limited time and place for partial reps, and I'll show you when, where and why to use them.

● Intelligence

Ok, here's where we go off the trail and delve into an area that almost all weightlifting systems ignore. Many people consistently train with compound exercises using progressive resistance—for a while. But then, several things typically start to happen. They get hurt—often more frequently as they age. They forget things. Then the slow decline begins. It's all because they didn't know how to train intelligently for a lifetime. Often, it's an issue of ego versus intelligence, with ego routinely winning with the young at heart. That typically results in injuries or no progress. I'll show you how to train intelligently so you reduce the likelihood of injury and chronic issues. I'll show you how 'instinctive training' is really just training without a plan, like meandering through a desert for years (and maybe seeing a mirage or two), and how to absolutely know what you need to do to keep progressing. In addition, I'll show you how those assistance exercises are the final key in turning you into a mutant among men.

Muscles & Their Function: What You Need to Know

Let's make sure you understand what the purpose of each of your muscles are before we go any further. I'm still amazed all these years later at how many people in the gym labor away for years without this basic knowledge. If you don't have this understanding you will never optimize the muscular physique that lies within. It allows you to unlock the code to muscular development.

You may see terms such as flexion, abduction, external rotation, etc. describing how muscles and joints function. We're not going to use those terms, since you won't remember them, and you probably don't care.

The table below presents the functions of each group of muscles (body part) in easy to remember concepts.

Body Part	Function	Typical Exercises
Abs	Moves your chest towards your waist, flexes the spinal column and lifts the ribs and moves them together.	Crunches, Reverse Crunches
Back	Pulls the shoulders down and backwards.	Chins, Rows
Biceps	Lifts and curls the arm and turns the wrist up.	Curls, especially Dumbbell Curls
Calves	Flexes the foot.	Calf Raises
Chest	Pulls the arms and shoulders across the front of the body.	Presses, Flys
Forearms	Curls the palm up and down.	Wrist Curls, Reverse Wrist Curls
Hamstrings	Curls the leg back (brings your foot to your butt).	Leg Curls
Quads	Extends and straightens the leg.	Leg Extensions, Squats, Leg Press
Shoulders	Rotates and lifts the arm to the	Presses, Laterals

Body Part	Function	Typical Exercises
	front, side, and rear.	
Traps	Raises the shoulders up.	Shrugs, Upright Rows
Triceps	Straightens the arm and turns the wrist down.	Presses, Pushdowns, Dips

Every movement you make in life is typically a combination of these functions.

For example, let's say you are eating a bowl of soup. You need to extend your arm forward (shoulders) and straighten it somewhat (triceps), perhaps turning your wrist slightly (forearm) to place the spoon in the bowl. Then, you curl your arm back up to your mouth (biceps and shoulders, again), perhaps bending your head down which lifts your shoulders slightly (traps). Even the simple act of eating soup involves your shoulders, biceps, triceps, forearm, and traps.

Here's one more example. Hang with me through this—I'll get to the point shortly.

Let's say you are standing and drop a pen you were holding.

You bend over, squat down, move your arm to the pen, pick it up and stand back up.

Here's what you just used:

Abs + Quads + Hamstrings + Calves + Triceps + Shoulders + Back + Biceps

Now, substitute a loaded barbell for the pen and you've got a deadlift. A compound, multi-joint exercise that works a hell of a lot of muscles in your body in one movement. This is why compound, multi-joint free weight exercises pack on muscle quicker than anything else known to man. If you consistently use these types of exercises in a progressive fashion and in an intelligent manner, you will become and remain a superman among men your age for most of your life.

Training Frequency

How many days per week should I workout? That's usually one of the first questions asked, and for good reason—it's vitally important in order to walk that tight rope between anabolism and overtraining.

Here's what you should do:

- **3-5 days per week works best.**

- **3 days per week** for those following a specific, heavy power lifting or sports strength program and for those following whole body workouts.

- **4 days per week** for most trainers who want to maximize muscle size via a one-week workout rotation, as recommended below. This is the one that most people should probably use and the one I've had the most success with.

- **5 days per week** for those with more time and more ability to recover and split their training sessions.

- **More than 5 days per week and you greatly increase your chance of being over-trained**; which means you'll actually get weaker and smaller. We don't want that.

Workout Scheduling

Now that you know how many days per week to work out, you need some guidelines on how to go about scheduling your workouts for those days. Here they are.

- **Try to give each body part at least 48 hours rest.**

- **Give yourself a day off after a quad workout.** Why? It's simple. Quads/glutes are the biggest muscle group, you should be doing squats as the basis of your quad workout, and squats cause a large systemic draining effect on your entire body. If you do a quad workout correctly (intensely) your system will be shot. Give it some rest after that.

- **Don't work the same body part two days in a row.** For example, if you are working chest today, then don't work delts or triceps tomorrow. You just worked them (indirectly) when you worked chest.

- **For each workout, train your muscles from largest to smallest.** This sequence optimizes energy expenditure by allocating your full energy to the larger muscles and allowing your remaining energy to be used for the smaller muscles. Follow this strategy unless you are attempting to correct a weak point or unless otherwise noted elsewhere in this system.

  The hierarchy of muscle groups, from largest to smallest is:

  1. Quads/Glutes
  2. Back
  3. Chest
  4. Traps
  5. Hamstrings
  6. Delts
  7. Triceps
  8. Biceps
  9. Calves
  10. Forearms
  11. Abs

So, for example, if you are going to train chest and triceps, you should train chest **THEN** triceps, and not triceps **THEN** chest. Pretty simple and effective, so stick to it.

- Good examples of a 4 day per week workout schedule, based on the guidelines above, include:

    o **Tues**: Chest/Delts/Abs

    o **Wed**: Quads

    o **Fri**: Arms/Calves/Abs

    o **Sun**: Back, Traps, Hamstrings

    o **Tues**: Arms/Calves/Abs

    o **Wed**: Quads

    o **Fri**: Chest/Back

    o **Sun**: Delts, Traps, Hamstrings

Training Volume

At this point, you know how many days per week to work out, and you know how to schedule those workouts. Now, it's just down to exercise selection and how many sets to do—training volume.

Proper training volume has always been a hotly debated topic, and like any political arena, there are the moderates and the extremists (high-volume vs. high intensity). Here's what I've seen works best:

● **For most individuals a moderate training volume will work best.** This equates to roughly 10-12 sets per large body part, and 8-10 sets per small body part. These are working sets and do not include warm up sets.

● **The systemic effect on your body includes not only your working sets, but your warm up sets as well.** Keep that in mind. Due to this, it's recommended that you record your warm up sets in your training log as well as your working sets. This is valuable information that can help you determine how much total training volume and system stress your body can take.

● **Suggested training volume, including warm up sets, per body part, from most volume to least:**

  o Quads: 15-20 sets

  o Back: 12-16 sets

  o Chest: 12-15 sets

  o Delts: 12-14 sets

  o Biceps/Triceps: 10-12 sets

  o Calves: 8-12 sets

  o Hamstrings: 8-10 sets

  o Abs/Forearms: 6-8 sets

● You'll notice that the suggested training volume for each body part roughly translates from the most volume for the largest muscle group to the least volume for the smallest muscle group. There are exceptions, though.

● The training volume for Delts is approximately the same as for Chest/Back, since the shoulder complex is composed of three distinct heads—front, side, rear. You want to look good from all angles, so we need to add some additional volume here so no one feels left out.

● Hamstrings are heavily involved with squats and leg presses, so we don't need to perform quite as many sets as we normally would. Of course, if your hamstrings are lagging, then you should add a couple more sets.

● **Your guiding precept on training volume should be to use the minimal number of sets that induce that body part to grow and no more.** You'll find that as you increase the intensity, the number of sets that you can effectively do decreases. You can train hard or you can train long, but you can't do both. Opt to train hard.

● The training routines offered in the workout section were not devised just for this book. They are actual battle-tested routines performed over the course of twenty years and adhere to the guidelines above. Master all the routines and you'll win the war.

Am I Over Trained?

It's very common to walk into any gym and notice that a lot of people are either under-training or over-training. If you follow the concepts in this book, you won't under-train. However, how do you recognize when you are over-trained?

Your level of training and progress is a composite of your training frequency, volume, intensity, rest, and nutrition. Get too much frequency, volume and intensity, or too little rest and proper nutrition and you'll end up in an over-trained state. You do not want this. Remember Newton's Law of Motion? I'll adapt it for our **Law of Physical Progress: a body in motion (progressing) tends to stay in motion.** You want to stay on a roll. That's why consistency is the most important principle. Over-training brings you to a complete and utter halt, and can sometimes move you backward. Yikes.

Here are the typical symptoms of over-training:

- Decreased exercise performance

- Decreased ability to achieve a muscle pump

- Excessive fatigue and lethargy

- Excessive muscle aches and joint pain

- Insomnia and restlessness

- Loss of appetite

- Elevated heart rate

- Frequent or lingering illnesses

- Decrease in lean body mass

- Agitation, mood swings, irritability and lack of focus

- Lack of motivation to train

I've found that the most reliable signs of over-training are a combination of excessive fatigue, fighting to achieve a pump, reduced appetite, a slight reduction in leanness, followed by general irritability.

If you find yourself in an over-trained state (or nearing one), do the following immediately:

1. **Increase the amount of sleep you are getting.**

2. **Increase the amount of protein you are eating.** Also, check your carbs. You may be eating too little.

3. **Completely change the exercises you use in each workout.**

Rep Ranges

So how many reps should you do for a set? The answer depends on what your goal is. If you're reading this book, then your goal should be to maximize muscular development. There are tried-and-true rep ranges for this (6-12 reps). But there are other rep ranges you shouldn't ignore either:

● **For mass, stick with 5-9 reps.**

● **To get at all muscle fiber types use the entire spectrum of ranges during your workout, anywhere from 5 to 25.** Good categories of ranges are 6-8, 8-12, 12-15, and 15+. Just remember the risk/reward ratio here—the lower you go, the more muscle mass and strength you will gain, but the higher the risk of injury. Conversely, the higher you go, the more muscle endurance you will gain (but less mass) with diminishing chance of injury. Know your body, and work your muscles through the spectrum of rep ranges that suit your goals and situation.

The table below summarizes reps ranges and their typical adaptation responses. Note that we are talking about "typical" adaptation responses—yours may vary slightly, and that's where the tracking system you use to record your workouts comes into play (I'll talk about that later).

Max Reps	Typical Adaptation Response
1-3	Pure strength
4-8	Mostly strength + some endurance
9-15	Strength + endurance
16-25	Some strength + endurance
25+	Muscular endurance + some cardiovascular endurance
100+	Cardiovascular endurance

Additionally, you may hear personal trainers, various books, or other systems talk about determining your one rep max (1RM) and basing your exercise reps on this value. This system does not rely on 1RM—however; it can be a useful barometer for determining how many reps you should be able to perform, if you are curious.

The table below provides an approximation of percentage 1RM to the number of reps equivalent:

% of 1RM	Reps
100%	1RM
90-99%	2-3
80-89%	4-6
70-79%	7-10
60-69%	11-15
50-59%	16-20

The 3:1, 2:1 and 1:1 Methods

Over time, I've noticed that there are several general methods, when used appropriately, that can help you make consistent progress (the 3:1 Method), encourage symmetry (the 2:1 Method) and reduce your chance of injury (the 1:1 Method). Intelligent use of these methods over a lifetime of weight training will further distance you from the average weight trainer.

3:1 Method

The purpose of this method is to allow muscle growth to continue in a linear fashion, while avoiding plateaus.

- **Rule: For every three similar workouts you perform, the next one should be radically different.**

- For example, let's say your bicep workout for the past three sessions consisted of barbell, dumbbell and preacher curls, in that order, for 10 total working sets. Your next workout should look nothing like that. A good alternative would be one-arm cable hammer curls, Zottman curls, and seated barbell curls, for 12 working sets. Notice that the first exercise (one-arm hammer curls) is a cable exercise (constant tension) done unilaterally, the second exercise is an unusual dumbbell movement, and the barbell curl is done last, in a seated position. The workout volume is also slightly increased. Radically different.

2:1 Method

The purpose of this method is to ensure that your body symmetry stays in balance, as well as to help you improve a body part that may be slightly lagging in progress.

- **Rule: When training multiple body parts in a single workout, for every two workouts that you begin with body part A, the next workout should start with body part B.**

- For example, if you train chest and shoulders in the same workout, you've probably noticed that you can't use as much weight on your shoulder pressing movements as you can if you worked shoulders either alone or first in the workout. Therefore, every third workout, start your chest/shoulder workout with shoulders. It will actually help your chest improve as well.

● Another example. Let's say you work quads and hamstrings in the same workout and your hamstrings could use some improvement, especially in relation to your quads (sound familiar?). Every third leg workout, start with hamstrings. Over time, you should notice a big improvement.

1:1 Method

The purpose of this method is to minimize your chance of injury.
Several exercises should not be performed two workouts in row, due to the stress they put on the spine, neck, elbows and knees.

● Change your foot and hand placement every other workout (more on this below).

● Don't perform extensions (skull crushers) two workouts in a row. Lying and seated E-Z bar and barbell extensions are notorious for placing a lot of strain on the inner elbow tendon.

● Don't perform hack squats two workouts in a row. Hack squats place a lot of strain on the knee joint. Give 'em a break every other week and you'll continue to progress on them at a much better rate in the long run.

The 3:1, 2:1 and 1:1 Methods

Weight Training Tips & Techniques

Follow these general guidelines in order to maximize your muscular potential and minimize your injury risk. The specific body part sections, which follow, will provide you with years of weight training insights, saving you lots of experimentation and allowing you to perform exercises in the most effective manner possible.

Using Free Weights & Machines

- **Free weights rule.** Think barbells and dumbbells. Not only will they make you stronger and bigger, they'll also make you a better athlete—at any age.

- **Machines can be useful when you need to take a break from your normal routine or when you are dealing with an injury.** Since machines provide a tracked, non-balancing system, they can be especially helpful when dealing with sore lower backs, tendon strains, etc. Just make sure that the track the machine has you performing doesn't directly affect the injured area—and get back to the free weights as soon as possible. You're not going to build a highly muscular and athletic body by using machines.

- **Compound, multi-joint movements should be the centerpiece of every workout.** These mass building exercises allow for the use of heavy weights. Hard work on these exercises typically produces the fastest muscle mass gains possible. In the body part sections below, you'll see the exercises categorized as **Key Exercises** and **Alternate Exercises**.

- **Key Exercises** are generally compound, multi-joint movements that will produce the greatest muscular effect on your body. They should comprise the vast majority of your exercise selections, and you should usually do these first, before selecting any of the alternate exercises.

- **Alternate Exercises** are useful as supplementary exercises, for providing mental and injury relief, and for breaking past plateaus. Just don't rely on them or use them too frequently.

Warming Up

- **Always warm up** before starting your workout. General stretching, including hanging from a chinning bar and moving your muscles through their full range of motion are always a good idea. Do it every workout—even if you are in a hurry. Oh, and if you're in a hurry, don't be surprised if you get injured. You have been warned.

- Perform at least one warm-up set for each exercise. Muscles don't react well to sudden surprises, especially with ungodly poundage.

Form & Range of Motion

- **Use a full range of motion**—almost all of the time. Partial reps are a valuable technique, but they should comprise a small portion of your overall training plan. Don't become a member of half-rep nation—unless you want half a physique. The full range of motion man will beat you every time. Two areas where you can always spot if someone doesn't perform full range movements are quads and back. More on this later.

- **Do not throw weights. You lift weights.** This means using your muscles to lift and lower the weight, and squeezing the hell out of it. Anybody can throw weights around. It takes courage to start with light weights, get the proper form and feel of the exercise, and slowly work your way up in poundage. In this case, the tortoise will always beat the hare. Always.

- **Again, use proper form.** Lift the weight. Don't add extraneous body movements into an exercise. Don't dip your body downward (even slightly) when curling, performing laterals or pushdowns—just pick a lighter weight and do it correctly. You might actually feel the muscle contract. And for god's sake, stay in your shoes. The only time your heel should come off the ground is when you are performing calf raises or some form of plyometric/explosive movement—not when you are doing front raises.

- **Squeeze your muscles during and between sets.** Along with proper form and controlled movements, you really need to squeeze the muscle(s) that you are working. How hard should you squeeze? As hard as you possibly think you can, and then even harder, as if the muscle is going to literally pop out of your skin. You would be surprised and how something as simple as squeezing your muscles extremely hard can make big differences in muscle density over the long term. You would be surprised at how many people don't do this.

● **If you're relatively young and use absolutely perfect form all the time, then you're not going to reach your full muscular potential.** There is a time and a place for looser form, using very heavy weights. Maximum muscle results from the correct use of perfect and loose form. In general, you'll always use perfect form for the majority of your workout (more than 50% of the time), but as you age, this percentage will continue to increase toward 100%. If you don't learn to do this, then both your injury potential and subsequent recovery time will increase.

● **Don't perform 1RM attempts at each workout.** In fact, don't try it every other workout either. You've probably seen countless guys (why is it always guys?) doing this week after week, month after month, etc. Then, they show up with shoulder pain ('cause they're not doing a 1RM on squats or dips, are they?) or some other injury. Wake up and grow up.

● **If you feel pain when doing an exercise, then don't do it.** This is your body putting up a big warning sign. Try to find another exercise for that body part that doesn't cause pain. Then, after several weeks, come back to that original exercise and see if you still have pain when performing it. If you do, you might want to go see a sports medicine doctor about that—and cross that exercise off your list for the foreseeable future.

● **If you strain a tendon or pull a muscle, the next time you work that body part keep the reps around 15.** If you are trying to rehab a chronic strain, do sets of 25-50 reps for that area—the blood that you flush into that area will help in the rehab.

● **Some exercises are difficult for some people to perform, due to body structure.** Tall guys always seem to have trouble squatting. People with wide clavicles (shoulders) and rib cages typically don't get the same results on bench presses as guys with barrel-shaped chests—but their shoulders grow like weeds. It's called physics and gives a leverage advantage/disadvantage to certain people. Use that knowledge to your advantage. Try substituting dumbbell presses for barbell presses, leg presses and hack squats for squats and front squats, etc. Don't get discouraged if you have some structural deficiencies. Almost everybody does. If you have problems squatting, you might just be a beast on deadlifts. Why do you think powerlifting competitions have three different lifts? It's the rare individual who is brutally strong on everything.

- **Be very careful with high-risk exercises**, which place certain body structures in precarious positions. In most cases, this means your shoulders. There is a reason why many sports organizations have banned their athletes from doing Behind the Neck Presses. Also, watch out for single dumbbell triceps extensions behind your head. One wrong move with heavy weights on those exercises could be the end of your lifting career. I've seen it—several times.

- **Stay within the natural range of motion that your body dictates.** Just because you saw Arnold in some magazine performing dumbbell flys where the dumbbells are touching the ground with his chest stretched all the way out does not mean that you can necessarily do the same. Maybe you can, maybe you can't. Use consistent stretching exercises to try to increase your range of motion—not exercises.

Placement of Hands and Feet

- The placement of your hands on a barbell and your feet on leg exercises are important variables to consider when working out over long periods. Let me give you an example. Let's say you perform 3 sets of 10 reps for 10 different exercises during your typical workout. That's 300 total reps per workout. If you work out three times per week, that's 900 reps for the week. If you do this week after week, month after month, with the same grip width and foot stance on your exercises, what do you think will happen?

- Imagine this. Let's say you walk in the grass between your front door and the mailbox about 900 times per week, always on the same path (evidently, you've got nothing else to do). The grass eventually erodes into dirt. Eventually, the dirt forms a rut. The same thing happens to your body, specifically your joints, tendons, and ligaments. Bye, bye shoulders, elbows and knees.

● By combining the 3:1 and 1:1 Methods with changes in the placement of your hands and feet (intra-workout or inter-workout), you greatly delay the formation of the "rut".

● Remember, there are always at least three different options for hand and foot placements: normal, narrow, and wide.

● Many people ask, "Where should I hold the bar?" Your normal hand position on a barbell can be determined by doing this—while standing, start swinging your arms at your sides. Now swing them right onto the bar. Yep, it's that simple. Just make a note of where your hand and fingers are in relation to the mark between the knurling on the bar. Now you know what your "normal" is.

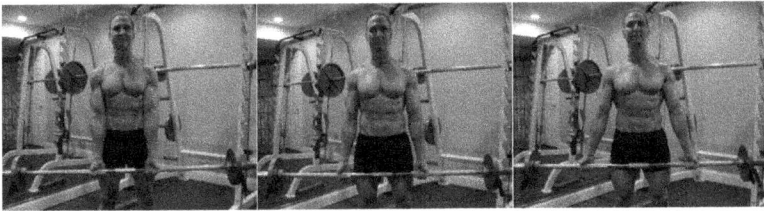

Narrow, Normal, and Wide grips on the barbell

● Your narrow grip is anything where your hands are closer than "normal". Use finger-widths and knurling marks on the bar to find comfortable and effective narrow grips for various exercises. Hint: they may differ across various exercises. Use the same process for the wide grip.

Getting Past Plateaus

● **If you are stuck at a plateau, try increasing the weight and lowering the reps for a couple workouts.** It may sound counterintuitive, but it typically works. After a couple weeks, you should be able to go back to where you hit the plateau and bust right past it.

● **Another technique that sometimes works is performing a few sets with an increased weight, but a limited range of motion.** However, make sure that you don't make a habit of this on the exercise, and that you always perform additional sets with full range of motion.

Stretching

● **Stretch consistently.** Treat stretching the same as your lifting. Do it before, during and after each exercise. You might be amazed at how flexible you become as your muscles grow.

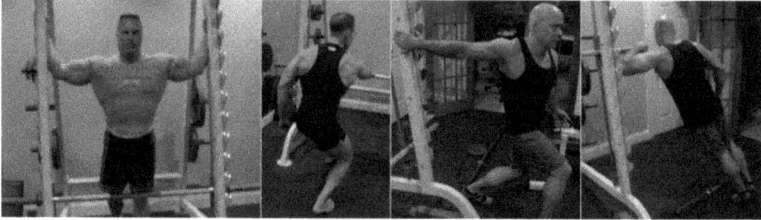

Stretching the chest, lats, biceps, and triceps

Wraps, Straps and Belts (oh, my!)

● **Ever see guys working out in the gym that always wear a weight belt? Don't do that.** About the only time you really should wear a weight belt is when you are performing heavy squats, deadlifts or standing overhead presses. Wearing a belt at other times will actually weaken the core muscles around your midsection since the belt is acting as a crutch. Let those core muscles get involved with all exercises—they'll get stronger and you'll feel better. You wouldn't use a crutch if you didn't have a problem walking on your leg, would you?

● As for other gym battle equipment, **try not to use knee or elbow wraps** unless you absolutely need to. And that means that you have a mechanical or injury issue with those joints and need to keep them secure and warm.

● **Wrist straps. Don't use them unless you are pulling on some mighty big weights.** Even then, try to perform a few sets without them. Automatically strapping on your wrist straps whenever you do back exercises, shrugs, and upright rows is a surefire way to limit your forearm strength and size. And please, don't wear them all the time, like when you are doing curls. You'll only look stupid.

Training Partners & Spotters

● **Try to find a training partner that's stronger than you.** This seems obvious, but I have to throw it out there. Over time, you should reach the strength level of your partner.

● **If you need to use a spotter, seek out a competent one**—otherwise, do another exercise, work out in a power rack, or don't use one at all. A bad spotter can actually injure you.

Unwritten Rules of the Gym

● **Don't speak to someone performing a set, especially if they are using heavy weight.** This causes distractions and can cause injury. Believe me, I've seen it numerous times. Someone will be shrugging and a "friend" wanders by and asks him if so-and-so has come in to work out. Shrugger turns his head and ends up not being able to move his neck/head properly for a couple days due to a muscle sprain. Gee, thanks. We're not being rude when we ask you to shut up, we just want to concentrate and not get hurt. Note, we are not dismissing the use of positive commentary ("come on, you can do it—just one more rep") when you do your set—just superfluous banter that can wait until the set is over.

● **Don't stand right in front of the dumbbell rack when you are exercising**, even if you are performing strip sets down the rack. Pick up your dumbbells and take two steps back. This will allow others to get at dumbbells on the rack in front of you. It is not your exclusive dumbbell rack.

● If you are using the squat rack to hold your barbell for barbell curls and someone wants to squat, remember the unwritten rules of the gym, give him the squat rack and pick up the bar off the floor. It's a squat rack, not a barbell curl holder. You might just add some additional muscle by picking up stuff off the floor.

● **Put your weights away when you are done.** Failure to do this shows a complete lack of respect for others who will use the equipment after you—and it shows what a true son-of-a-bitch you probably are in other aspects of life. The next person might not want to leg press 700+ pounds—but on the other hand, they might want to curl 135lbs and not your measly 65.

● **If you are using a piece of equipment and need to go to the water fountain, bathroom, etc.,** place a towel, water bottle, etc on or beside the equipment to indicate that someone is using it. Be quick—don't leave for five or more minutes, come back to find someone else on the equipment and say, "hey, I was using that."

● **If in doubt, ask if someone is using the equipment you are eyeing.** They may have just popped away to the water fountain or to find another plate.

● **Don't parade around the gym if you have big arms, delts or chest, but no legs.** Holster your guns, 'cause somebody is probably moving around with some serious treads. Huge, muscular legs deserve utmost respect, since we all know what kind of torture, sacrifice and pain it probably took to get those things. They don't come cheap or easily. Remember—your upper body workouts are nothing compared to serious leg sessions.

The Strongest Muscles

● Finally, get it through your head right now. **Fat does not equate to big—as in muscular big.** If you're fat (and you know if you are), then you really need to tighten your diet and get intimate with cardio work (5-6 days per week, 30-45 minutes per session depending on how much fat you need to lose). Here's the general rule of thumb to check if you are fat or not—hold your arms above your head and look in the mirror. Can you see your serratus muscles (those finger-like muscles at the side of your ribcage, connecting your lats and abs)? If you can't, then it's time for a tighter diet and more cardio. Otherwise, you're good to go. Stop fooling yourself and get really big, the lean way. It's been said many times before, and it's true. A lean 16" arm will appear much larger than a fat 19" arm. Think about that.

- Larry Scott, the first Mr. Olympia, astutely noted that about **80% of the dumbbells in any gym get used regularly, while the top 20% in weight typically collect dust**, regardless of the actual weights. In other words, if your gym has dumbbells going up to 150lbs, I bet those 130s, 140s and 150s don't get used a lot. You need to break through this mental barrier (and oh, it does exist) that manifests itself on the dumbbell rack and throughout your travails in and out of the gym (with the mirror, scale, your waist, strength, etc.).

- Although genetics play a large part in your ultimate metamorphosis, **those with intelligent training and big hearts full of desire often surpass those with superior genetics and half-ass training.** Cast iron has a way of finding out how much heart you have. Remember, when your mind fails, your heart will take over.

- Finally, **the mirror is your worst friend**. While the uninformed may think that your constant gaze of yourself is nothing more than a narcissistic delusion of grandeur, you should be using the mirror as both a friendly tool to verify correct exercise performance and as a method of analyzing your weaknesses. Be honest. Accept your flaws and do something to correct them.

Abs

Moves your chest towards your waist, flexes the spinal column and lifts the ribs and moves them together.

Key Exercises	Reverse Crunches (Flat, Incline, Hanging), Crunches, Twists
Alternate Exercises	Incline Sit-Ups, Leg Raises, Side Bends

General Tips

● People with great abs have done two things: worked their abs consistently hard and know how to eat properly to maintain low body fat levels. It's the second one that trips up almost everyone. The diet section in this book will help you with that.

● What's the biggest mistake when working abs?—working your hip flexors hard without working your abdominals at that same intensity. Most people don't even realize they are doing this. The section below on Leg Raises and Reverse Crunches will help you with this.

● **The greater the range of motion you can achieve when performing abdominal work, the better.** This is one reason why Swiss Balls have become so popular—they provide you with a greater range of motion, since you start with a curved spine and stretched abs before you crunch.

● Try this experiment: if you usually perform 6 sets for abs, do all of your ab sets with reverse crunches. Do this for a couple weeks. Notice where you feel ab soreness and how your abs appear—no worse than if you did regular crunches, huh? That's because reverse crunches really improve one of the weakest areas of your body—bringing your lower pelvis up toward your chest. Strengthening that area is a win-win all the way around. Your abs will look great, your posture will improve, and your lower back will thank you.

- If you can perform multiple sets of 25+ reps of weighted hanging crunches, then consider yourself awarded the PhD in Abdominals. Dr. Abdominal. You the man.

- **Always stretch your abs after finishing your ab workout.** They're just like any other muscle group, and you stretch those, don't you? One of the best ab stretches is to lie face down on the floor, press your hips into the floor and slowly rise your upper torso up, using your forearms as support. Hold that stretch and keep those hips flat on the floor.

Leg Raises and Reverse Crunches

- There is a big difference between leg raises and reverse crunches. Leg raises primarily work your hip flexor muscles, while reverse crunches remove those muscles from the movement and isolate your abdominals. Most people are just performing leg raises, and will get great hip flexors, but wonder why their lower ab strength just isn't there. All reverse crunches start with your legs bent at a 90-degree angle at the knees. From there, using only lower abdominal strength, try to bring your lower torso toward your chest. Think of it as shortening your midsection, from the bottom up. It's not that big of a movement, but if you do it correctly, you should feel a strong contraction and eventual lactic acid burn emanating from your nether regions. Reverse crunches are the king of abdominal movements. Show me a person who can perform lots of reps of hanging reverse crunches with weight, and I'll show you someone with exceptional abdominal strength.

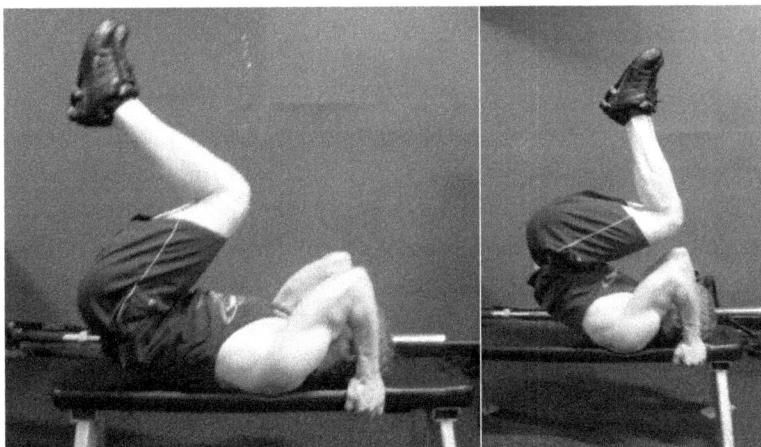

The Reverse Crunch—start and end positions

- Once you master reverse crunches on a flat surface, start doing them on an incline. Over time, increase the angle of incline until you are performing them hanging. Once you master hanging, use the medicine ball technique below for additional resistance.

- You can add resistance to your reverse crunches by squeezing a medicine ball between your lower thighs at the knee area. Use heavier and heavier medicine balls as you get stronger.

- Just because reverse crunches are so good of an abdominal movement, doesn't mean you shouldn't perform leg raises as well. We all need strong hip flexors. Just keep your focus on the reverse crunches and use leg raises as a secondary exercise.

Machine Abdominal Exercises

- When using machines to work your abs, remind yourself of caveat emptor—let the buyer beware. Even if you adjust the machine to best suit your frame, many ab machines can still play havoc with your lower back. Pay attention each time you do machine exercises for your abs. Does your lower back feel stiff/sore or hurt the next day or so? If you notice this trend, stick with body movements for abs (maybe with some free weight assistance), which is always the best option.

Side Bends

● You'll see lots of people performing this type of exercise, typically with dumbbells. Just be aware that the abdominal muscles at your sides tend to grow extremely easily, since it's not a normal body movement in everyday life. Perform side bends with high reps (25-50) and different types of apparatus (dumbbells, barbell, cables, bands) to see what kind of results you get.

Sit-ups & Crunches

● When performing any type of sit-up or crunch, don't put your hands behind your head and use them to assist you in performing the exercise. What this typically evolves into is some type of weird, bastardized head/neck movement, with very little ab work happening. Instead, make your hands into fists and keep them next to your temples at the side of your head. No hand involvement means more ab recruitment.

Twists

● **Ab twists are underrated.** Performing high-rep (25-100) sets of twists using a broomstick will do wonders for bringing out your intercostals and obliques. Combine that with reverse crunches, pullovers and low back work and you just built yourself the best shock absorber ever invented.

Wood Chops

● If you've watched just about any typical personal trainer at a gym, you've no doubt seen them take their clients through this exercise, like automatons building cars at a GM plant. What they are trying to do is build their client's internal obliques and all the muscles of the core. The trainer may even throw out the term du jour of 'functional training' as a reason for this. If you do chop wood to heat your home frequently, or load/unload packages onto your UPS/FedEx truck, then yes, this is functional training for you. If you follow the core tenets in this book— heavy, compound movements with free weights, especially with standing exercises (squats, deadlifts, presses, rows), your core will be stronger than any amateur wood chopper out there.

Chest

Pulls the arms and shoulders across the front of the body.

Key Exercises	Barbell Presses (Flat and Incline), Dumbbell Presses (Flat and Incline), Dips, Dumbbell Flys
Alternate Exercises	Decline Presses, Smith Machine Presses, Pec Dec Machine, Cable Crossovers

General Tips

● Chest is undoubtedly, along with biceps, the most popular and frequent body part worked in the gym. Unfortunately, it's also where egos reign and chest development suffers. Always keep two things in mind when working chest—don't over-train it, and don't let your ego pick the weight you use or dictate your form.

● **Try to alternate starting your chest workouts with incline and flat presses.** Always starting with flat presses can hamper your efforts to build that elusive upper chest. In fact, for a couple months, try starting all your chest workouts with an incline press to see how your upper chest responds. This is also why decline presses are not recommended, unless you are into building some droopy looking pecs.

● **For individuals with barrel-shaped ribcages, barbells will probably be the way to go for presses.** For those with wide and somewhat shallow ribcages, dumbbells will probably be more effective (especially for inclines) in activating the pecs and reducing the involvement of those Delts which always want to take over. You'll also find that handling heavy dumbbells for pressing is a real challenge that helps to muscularize your upper torso.

● **Don't get caught up in doing the same rep scheme with presses time after time.** Additionally, don't get trapped in the game of doing a one-rep max on bench presses each workout, or even every other workout. Save that for maybe once every 8 weeks. Mix it up a bit. Work through various rep ranges and get strong in all of them. Your chest development will significantly improve by doing this.

- **Pullovers with a dumbbell are a great way to stretch the pecs**, while working the entire shoulder and upper back structure. They also make a perfect transition movement between chest and back, since they activate the serratus and lats—great for a push-pull routine of chest/back.

- **Make sure you stretch your chest between sets.** Hang from a chinning bar, stretch your pecs between a doorway, Smith machine or other equipment.

- **Decline presses are useful occasionally, particularly when your bench presses hit a plateau**. Since most trainers are able to decline press more weight than either flat or incline, they can help you mentally and physically handle more weight on the bar. Do this for a couple weeks and see what happens to your flat bench--but don't make decline pressing a regular part of your chest workout. There is something much more effective…

- **Dips are much more effective than decline presses**, since they activate many more muscle groups (pecs, delts, triceps, traps, and even abs). Dips are like squats for the upper body. That's why about the same number of people do dips as squat—and just like squats, dips for the pecs require you to go deep into the dip. They're hard work but highly effective, especially when you start attaching weight to your body for them. The difference between maximizing dip effectiveness for your pecs versus triceps is depth and body angle. For pec dipping, you want to go low (to stretch the pecs) and have your body leaning forward (to contract the pecs through a fuller range of motion). Tuck your chin into your chest as well.

- **If you don't already have pretty good muscle mass on your pecs, don't spend time using the cable crossover**. It's not a mass building movement. If you don't have mass, why are you doing it? Stick with the barbells, dumbbells and dips. Cable crossovers are for advanced trainers with good pectoral mass who are trying to etch in final muscle cross-striations. It's like applying that final coat of stainless steel to your superstructure.

- **Don't forget about old-fashioned push-ups**—they are a great athletic movement that are also a perfect warm-up exercise for your chest workout. Do them on a decline for even greater intensity.

The Bench Press: King of the Jungle

- **Most people don't know how to bench effectively.** They start with incorrect foot placement, where their lower legs and feet are angled back so only the toes of the shoe are in contact with the floor. This helps to create excessive arch in the back, coupled with bouncing the bar off their chest, all in order to get those two or three reps up. It's an ungodly contortion, which only facilitates shoulder issues and under-developed pectorals. I've seen countless guys "benching" 300-400lbs this way, carrying around fat pecs that are no bigger than their calves. Let me tell you this—if you are pressing 300-400lbs for 6+ reps for multiple sets with correct form, your chest should be massive. You should be able to sit something on it.

- A correct bench press has the following characteristics—feet flat on the floor (there is one exception to this that I'll discuss below) with lower legs perpendicular to the floor, a slight arch in the chest with shoulders pinched back and down. Your grip on the bar should be very tight. Don't bounce the bar off your chest. You should feel mostly chest working, with some front delt and triceps (not too much). If you feel too much triceps, move your grip a little wider. If you feel too much front delt, concentrate on getting those shoulders back (pinch the shoulder blades together).

- Even with absolutely spot-on form, some individuals may still have difficulty getting their pecs to grow, usually at the expense of their front delts. The bench press (flat or incline) is kind to those with narrow clavicles and barrel-shaped ribcages. They have a body born to bench. Those of us with wide shoulders and wide, but shallow ribcages have to use a few tricks to try to even the playing field.

- Individuals with wide clavicles and narrow rib cage structures often find it hard to reduce the involvement of their shoulders in a bench press movement. For these people (and you know who you are), presses on the Smith machine may produce more results, since it will allow you to set and retain the shoulders back/down position you need to maximize pectoral involvement, without having to include the added involvement of bar stability which can easily knock you out of position. Try it and see what happens.

What to do when your Bench Press gets Stuck

● **When your bench press hits a plateau, the power rack becomes your best tool for breaking past that barrier.** You'll need a good power rack with pins that you can insert for full effectiveness of this technique. If your power rack only allows you to set a single height bar, you can still use this method but you won't be able to get the static contraction effect against a top set of pins. This technique uses partial movements (I told you there is a time and place for this) in order to increase your muscular power and prepare your body for handling heavier weights on the bench press.

● You are going to use three positions in the power rack—just touching your chest, mid-range (this is just below your sticking point), and lock-out. Start with the pins set so the bar just barely touches your chest. Set the upper pins about six inches higher. Load the bar with a weight you can perform full-range for about six reps. Now, get under the bar at the low position, and drive the bar forcefully into the upper pins (or about a foot up if you don't have upper pins) and hold it there for two seconds. Do this for three sets of five reps. Then, adjust the bottom pins so they are just below your sticking point and the upper pins six inches above that. Keeping the same weight on the bar, repeat the same explosive movement you did for the lower pin setting. You'll find the weight is much harder to handle in this position and much harder to hold against the upper pins for two seconds. This is the money position. After three sets of that, reset the pins so that they hold the bar about three inches below your total lockout height. You don't need upper pins for this lock-out position. Here, you are going to explode the bar up into full lockout. You should be using a weight that is at least 20% more than your 1RM on the bench—in any case, it needs to be heavier than anything you can bench for one rep. Keep using this technique any time you hit a plateau on the bench press.

● Don't forget—the three best exercises (other than benching) to increase your bench press are pushdowns, lying barbell extensions, and pulldowns behind the head. These three exercises build the muscles that help push that weight up (triceps and the lats—the lats are strongly involved in the first few inches of the bench press).

Incline Pressing

● There is much debate and disagreement over the most effective angle of incline to use—should it be 30°, 40°, or (gasp!) even 50°? Here's the answer. It depends. It depends on your body mechanics, set by your structure, arm length, etc. Here's how to find the answer for you. You are going to use either a barbell or dumbbells. You are going to do 20 sets of 10 of incline presses all at one specific angle that you pick. (If you are using a barbell, set it in a power rack and use an adjustable bench.) Yeah, that's a lot, but we want you to see where you are getting a pump, where the blood is flowing easily, and also, where you get sore the next day or two (or three) from this. Don't plan on doing any other exercises that day. We want to isolate the number of variables of this experiment you are performing on your body so that you know the exact relationship between angle and result. Is your chest filling with blood beyond belief? What about your shoulders? How involved are they? Are your shoulders affected equally as your chest? Think about these answers. A couple weeks later, do the same experiment, but at a different angle. Compare your results. Eventually, you should be able to determine the optimal angle that affects your chest. For me, 40° works best—nothing lower pumps my upper chest as much, and anything higher involves my front delts too much. After you find your answer, always remember—do what is most effective, not what you can handle the most weight with.

● **A good technique to use if your incline pressing hits a plateau is to lower the angle of attack temporarily.** This will allow you to handle a little more weight. In a couple weeks, go back to your normal angle and you should be able to go past that plateau.

● **Try incline presses with dumbbells using a neutral grip**, where your palms face each other. This is a move popularized by European weight lifters decades ago that provides a little different feel and contraction than normal dumbbell presses. At first, you'll find you won't be able to use as much weight, but as you acclimate to the movement, the weights will go up and so will your pecs.

● As you'll discover below, an effective way to work your upper chest is to keep your elbows in line with your shoulders. Typically, when doing incline presses, you'll find your elbows at about a 45° angle to your body. This is fine most of the time for most people. But you may want to try keeping your elbows high, up in line with your shoulders, in order to gauge the effectiveness of this type of movement. A good way to do this with dumbbells is to press them up while keeping your pinkie finger slightly higher than your thumb.

When to Use the Smith Machine

● The best uses of the Smith Machine for working chest are for when you want to go heavy but don't have a partner/spotter handy, for working past plateaus using the power rack technique described above, floor pressing, and for bench pressing to the neck. Otherwise, stick with barbells and dumbbells for your pressing.

● **Floor presses are a long forgotten method of bench pressing.** Bill Pearl describes the effectiveness of this exercise using a barbell in his seminal tome, *Keys to the Inner Universe*. Since it's hard to get a barbell into this position without the help of at least one partner, the Smith Machine becomes an excellent alternative. What you are going to do is lie down on the floor under the Smith Machine bar. When you bring the bar down, your elbows will contact the floor, allowing you to pause and then drive the bar up to lockout. This partial movement is good for working through the sticking point of the bench and learning to drive the weight up from a complete stop.

● **The Smith Machine is an effective upper pec builder**, especially when doing bench presses to the neck and high incline presses.

● **Smith Machine bench presses to the neck need to be done precisely**—otherwise, your shoulders are going to rebel against you. Done improperly, this exercise has a huge danger factor. Don't do this if you have any pre-existing shoulder issues. This was a favorite exercise that Larry Scott used to build his upper pecs, as described in *Loaded Guns*. There are three keys to performing this exercise properly; 1) pick a weight that you can do at least six reps with—anything heavier than this is just too dangerous for your shoulders; 2) lower the weight slowly, under control to your throat area; 3) keep your elbows high and your hands at a 45° angle on the bar—your upper arms should be in line with your shoulders. You should feel an extreme stretch across your upper pec area when the bar is near your throat. If you are using a Smith Machine, make sure you set the safety pins so that you don't get killed if something goes awry. You can also do this exercise in the power rack or on a regular bench press.

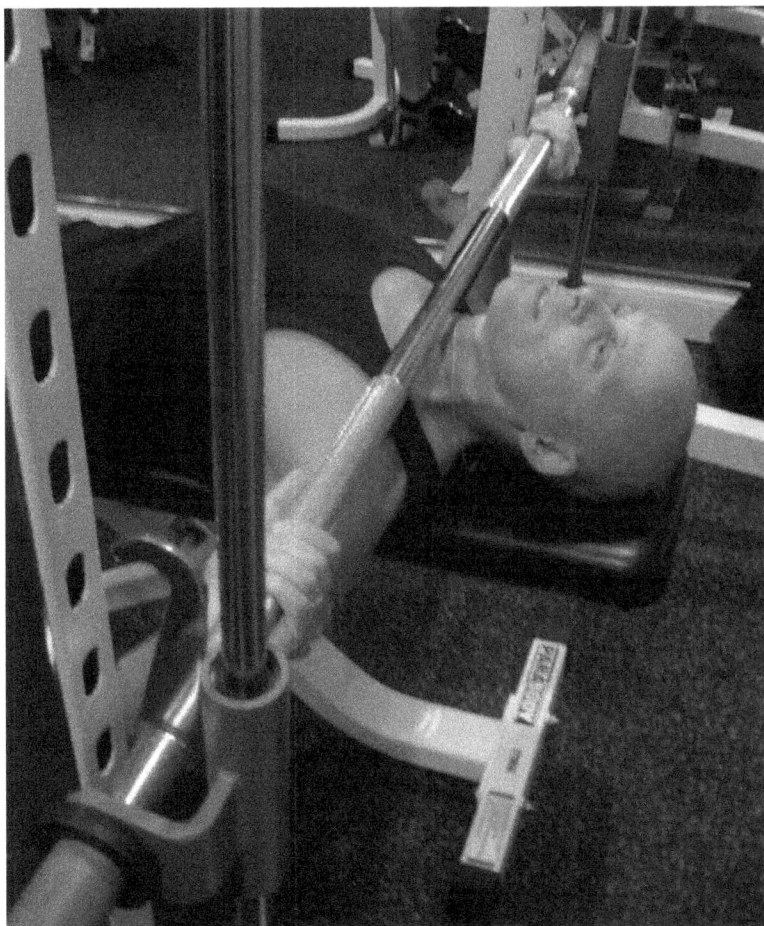

Smith Machine Bench Press to the Neck

- **The Smith Machine is good for performing barbell incline presses at many different angles**, something fixed incline benches don't allow. One useful angle is a high incline set at 50°. You'll feel a lot more front delt involvement at this angle, but you'll also notice with continued use how this exercise helps ties together your upper pec/delt tie-ins. You can also perform high incline presses in a power rack for greater intensity.

Fly Movements

- **When performing flys, perform flys.** Don't perform some inverted L-shaped movement that is halfway between a fly and a press. Flys are meant to stretch and contract the pecs through their natural range of motion. Set them free. You want a wide, sweeping arc. You want your elbow angle to remain constant. It's been said a million times, but it's a great analogy—act like you are hugging a tree, a big tree. I like to think that when you do flys correctly, you are hugging a big pot of gold that you've discovered.

- If the outer portion of your chest needs attention—if it doesn't have that squared off look to the pecs—other than using a slightly wider grip on barbell presses, you can perform your flys with a partial motion where you only come halfway up, tense, then lower and repeat. The pecs never get a chance to relax (like at the top of a fly) with this method.

- **Unless you have some type of shoulder problem, do dips instead of decline dumbbell flys.** There is nothing that a decline dumbbell fly can do that dips can't. Dips will put a whole lot more muscle on you than those flys will—in faster time. And they'll give you better shape. So, let the amateurs do the decline flys—you do the dips.

- **Effective cable crossovers can be performed several ways**, depending on the arc of motion—low (dip-like), chest-high (standard flys), upward (pec minor activation), or bent-over (simulates using rings).

- **Other than cable crossovers, cable flys (incline, flat, decline) are pretty much useless**, even with the advantages of continuous tension. Stick with dumbbells. They'll never let you down.

● Most gyms have a Pec Deck machine—it's a useful movement for providing maximum resistance at the peak contraction point on the fly movement. However, yet again, most lifters reduce the effectiveness of this exercise by not setting the seat height correctly and leaning their body forward in order to complete the rep. Most importantly, stay back against the pad, especially during the all-important peak contraction when your hands are almost touching. Only introduce forward torso movement after you can't complete another rep in strict form. As for seat height, you'll need to play around with different settings. Multiple seat heights are useful as they hit your pecs in slightly different areas. Experiment and note the effects.

● **You can also perform Pec Deck flys with one arm at a time.** Not only does this automatically increase intensity, but is also increases the range of motion slightly, allowing you to bring your hand a little further across your chest, since there is no opposing object to get in the way. This is about the only way you can effectively perform a unilateral fly movement with substantial weight.

Chest

Back

Pulls the shoulders down and backwards.

Key Exercises	Deadlifts, Chins, Bent-over Barbell Rows, T-Bar Rows, Seated Cable Rows, One-Arm Dumbbell Rows
Alternate Exercises	Lat Pulldowns, Hyperextensions

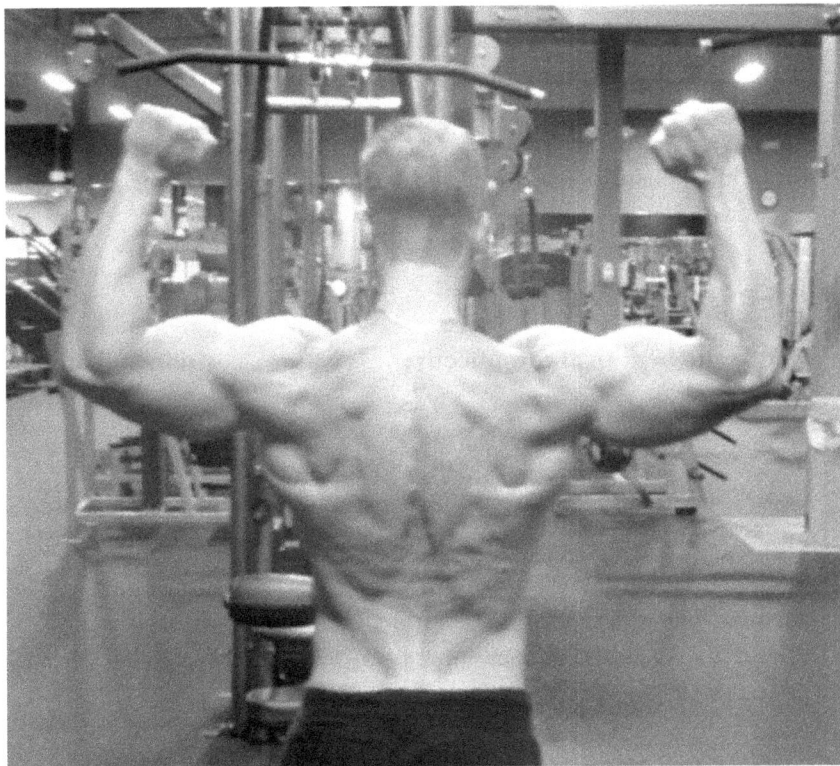

General Tips

● Why don't most people have nice, muscular, V-shaped backs tapering down to their waist? Three reasons: poor exercise selection, incorrect form, and perhaps a wide waist due to dietary issues. Read on to see how to get the V-shape.

- You can pick out the weight trainers in every gym who don't perform a full range of motion on their back movements—they're the ones that don't have a distinct V-taper. You just can't build an impressive V-taper without performing full-range back movements.

- **If you could only pick two back exercises to do, chins and barbell rows are it.** Oh, and deadlifts. That's three. Just remember, row, row, row your back and it will grow, grow, grow.

- **The general rules are: Chins/Pulldowns for width, rows for thickness.**

- Since the back is such a large collection of interconnected muscles, it responds well to volume and variety (exercises, grips, and rep ranges). Use that knowledge to your advantage.

- Remember, building a massive back and legs gets you two-thirds of the way to your ultimate muscular size.

Bent-over Rows

- **The key to bent-over row effectiveness is torso position and arching of the back.**

- You need to bend over so that your upper torso is about parallel to the floor if you want to work your lats fully on this exercise. That probably means you need to reduce the weight (swallow your pride) at first, to burn this form into your motor neurons. If you see guys standing at a 45° angle (or higher), using a good bit of weight, they are probably doing one of two things—working their upper back/traps, or not knowing what they are doing.

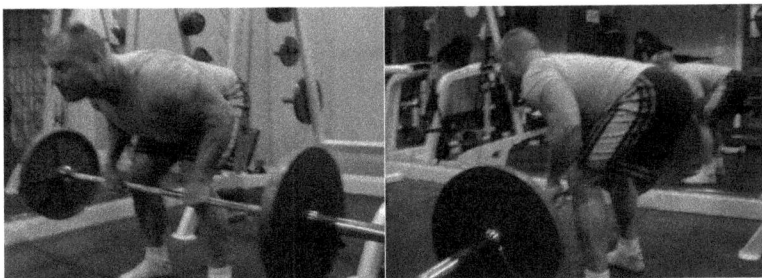

Correct form during the mid-point of bent-over rows

- After you get your torso in the correct position, make sure that you have a slight arch in your back. Failure to do that can result in lower back issues, as well as limiting your range of motion and contraction strength. You are trying to pull those elbows as far back (in this case, high) as possible. When you are arched correctly, think of each lat as a fan that you are trying to squeeze together.

- **Try different grip widths** as well as where you pull the bar to—to the navel, to the lower pec, to the nipples and higher. Feel how each pull target affects the result.

Chins & Pulldowns

- Do chins correctly. That means doing a full rep. That means going all the way down to a dead hang. That's not an easy thing to do for most, since it represents another pride-swallowing moment. Those who concentrate on lowering themselves under control to this position, then pulling themselves all the way up will be rewarded with a nice, wide back. You'll need some new shirts.

- If you can't perform a full rep of chins, start by using a bench to get yourself into the full contracted chin position and slowly lower yourself to a dead hang. Perform 3-5 of these for each set. If you want to get stronger on chins, you can use the same technique with a dipping belt and some plates hanging from your waist.

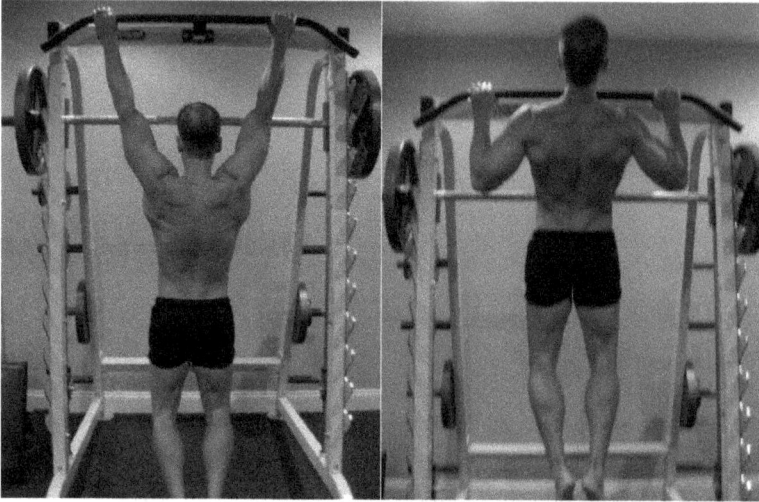

From dead hang to full contraction—a perfect chin

● **Variety of grip is essential for chins and pulldowns**. Use every type of pulldown attachment available to you. Use wide, narrow, neutral and reverse grips on chins. You don't have to change grips every set or even within your workout—but make sure you change grips at least from workout to workout.

Perfecting Pulldowns

● **Don't lean too far back when doing pulldowns to the front—** otherwise, you might as well just do seated cable rows since that's what you are changing the exercise into.

● Most gyms have poorly designed equipment for performing pulldowns to the rear. That's because the pulldown apparatus is optimized for pulling to the front. What you want is a straight vertical line from where the cable starts down, right to the back of your head/neck. If you face the machine, what typically happens is that you have to lean slightly forward to get the bar pulled down behind your head. This creates a sub-optimal movement when pulling to the rear. If you find yourself in this situation, try sitting backwards, facing away from the machine. Usually, that will put the cable in the correct vertical position for pulling straight down.

- Of all variations of pulldowns, reverse-grip pulldowns require the strictest form to produce the greatest results. You want your upper body to be as close to vertical when doing this type of pulldown. You also want to pull the bar down to mid-chest level (no further) and squeeze for ultimate results. Combine that with a full extension to dead-hang level and you have perhaps the perfect pulldown exercise.

Deadlifts

- **Deadlifts are like dark chocolate and red wine.** Performed correctly and in moderation, they are a wonderful, superior mass building movement almost unsurpassed. Overused, or done incorrectly and they can ruin you. First, you have to get your form correct, right from the start. You need a solid mechanical foundation upon which to add weight. Second, always remember you are not a powerlifter and are not competing in a powerlifting meet in the gym. There really isn't any good reason to go below five reps on each set (unless you are a competitive powerlifter—then go for it). Choose your weights wisely. If your form is not locked into the movement after a few warm-up sets, stop and move to another exercise. This one can come back to bite you quickly.

- **Deadlifts build quads.** That's half of the movement. Which doesn't mean it's part one of the movement...

- **Deadlifts are a compound exercise with a single, explosive movement.** Think about that. Don't make this exercise into a frightening two-stage booster shot straight up your spine. You are pushing the floor away from you with your quads at the same time you are pulling up and back with your back. Your arms are just along for the ride.

Hyperextensions vs. Good Mornings

- Aside from deadlifts, hyperextensions and Good Mornings are the two best exercises to develop your lower back (spinal erectors). What's the difference between the two? For most people, it's a little easier to injure yourself with Good Mornings, due to excessive rounding of the lower back, but you can use much more resistance on this exercise. The only thing you need to watch out for with hyperextensions is hyperextension—that is, over-arching of your lower back as you rise up.

This exercise should really be re-named back extensions. Let's leave the 'hyper' alone.

- Try super-setting sets of abs with sets of hyperextensions. This combo will really work your core, as well as stretching your abs while you work your lower back, and vice versa.

- What about the back extension machines found in most gyms? Give them only a passing glance, except if you are recovering from a low back injury—then, they become valuable for performing high-rep (15-25) back extensions for low intensity, blood-pumping, recovery-inducing work.

Lower Lats

- **The key to bringing out your lower lats is deadlifts and one-arm dumbbell rows.** Show me someone who has weak or non-existent lower lat development and I'll show you someone who doesn't do heavy deadlifts. When you are pulling a heavy weight from the floor, your entire lat, from top to bottom insertion will be working at full capacity. There just isn't any way around that. However, if you want to increase your lower lat development even further, then add in specialized one-arm dumbbell row work after your deadlifts.

- **One of the keys to lower lat development is range of motion**, especially with one-arm dumbbell rows. You need to lower the dumbbell to a dead hang, and then move the dumbbell slightly forward to increase the stretch further.

- **Reverse-grip pulldowns will also help to develop the lower lat area**, although not to the extent as deadlifts and one-arm dumbbell rows. It's essential that you use a full range of motion for this—all the way up to a dead hang, followed by a pull with your elbows so that the bar touches your lower chest area.

- So there you have it—deadlifts + one-arm dumbbell rows + reverse-grip pulldowns = ultimate lower back development.

Machine Rows

● **Machine rows are useful when you have a lower back injury** and need stabilization or when you need a brief change from your normal routine. Otherwise, relegate them to the seldom-used pile.

Pullovers

● **Pullovers are a great exercise to help tie everything together**—lats, intercostals, pecs, and shoulders. Bonus—if you are young (teenager or very early twenties) then pullovers may help to increase your rib cage size, since your connective tissue may still be pliable. The bigger the rib cage, the bigger the foundation you have to build a massive upper body structure.

● If you still have access to an old chain-driven Nautilus pullover machine (are there any still around?), then this is the best device ever made for performing pullovers. Otherwise, your options are dumbbells or a barbell. I would recommend using a dumbbell.

● When performing dumbbell pullovers, the biggest mistake I see is guys using too much weight and not lowering their hips at full dumbbell extension. You need to drop your hips the same time as you extend the dumbbell over your head, keeping your shoulder blades firmly planted across the bench. Inhale as you lower the dumbbell and dip your hips, and forcefully exhale as both rise to the start position. If you can do this with a 100+ lb dumbbell for high reps, then you are a better man than I.

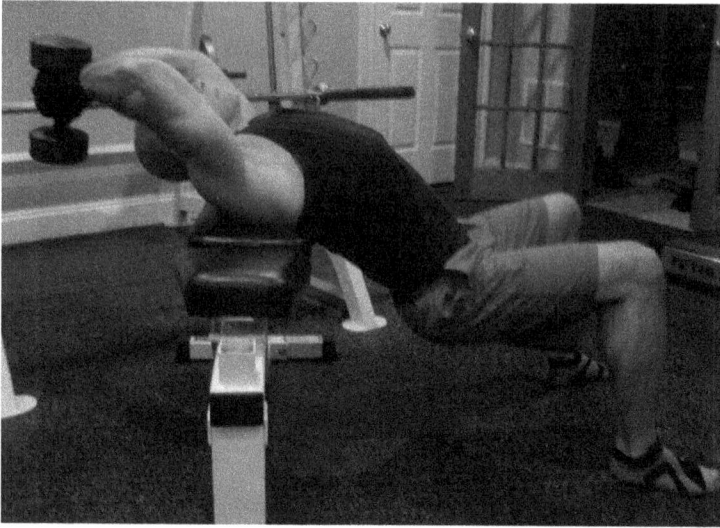

This is a correct pullover—hips lowered, back arched, ribcage up, extending arms back

Seated Cable Rows

● **The key to seated cable rows is at the beginning and end of the movement.** At the beginning, make sure your lats are stretched, but don't lean forward excessively—you just want the lats under tension. At the end, make sure that you pull the bar/handle to your body (not a foot in front of your body), and end with your torso in an upright or with a slight lean back—with the emphasis on 'slight'. Don't turn this into a rocking exercise.

T-Bar Rows

● **Effective T-Bar rowing shares the same concepts as Bent-over Barbell Rows**—correct torso position (near parallel to the floor) with a slight back arch.

● **Try using 25lb plates on the T-Bar**, instead of the typical 45lb plates. Of course, a happy medium would be 35lb plates, if your gym has them. The smaller plates will allow you to pull your elbows a little further back, giving you a greater range of motion. Of course, with the lighter plates, you'll need more of them, which means the laws of physics and fulcrums come into play...

Shoulders

Rotates and lifts the arm to the front, side, and rear.

Key Exercises	Military Presses (Barbell and Dumbbell), Arnold Presses, Dumbbell Lateral Raises (Front, Side, Rear), Rear Delt Machine/Reverse Pec Dec
Alternate Exercises	Presses Behind the Neck

General Tips

● Your Delts represent the start of the ideal classical Greek 'X' frame, and are one-third of that trifecta, including abs and calves. Delts are also the only body part that is visible from all angles. Think about that. You can't hide poor Delts. Get big Delts, carved abs, and well-developed calves and your fan base will grow.

● Always start with a pressing movement if your goal is mass. Then follow with laterals. If you feel yourself hitting a plateau on presses, try performing them last in your routine—but try to perform the same weight as before. You may surprise yourself the next time you work them first.

● Use a full range on shoulder presses. Don't stop lowering the weight at the top of your head. Build up your shoulder flexibility and lower the weight as far as you comfortably can. I lower the barbell to my collarbone and the dumbbells until they lightly touch my shoulders. That's what you can do when you stretch every day.

● Show me a person who has larger rear delts than front delts and I'll show you a freak. Due to the over-emphasis in gyms on pressing movements in lieu of posterior chain pulling movements, the front head of the delt always overpowers that rear head. To bring up the rear head, try performing rear laterals immediately after your presses. You might also want to perform 10 sets of 10 reps of rear laterals every couple shoulder workouts. You might like the results and your rotator cuff and labrum will remain structurally sound.

● Side and rear lateral machines just beckon you to employ drop-sets and 21s as shocking techniques—something not as easily done with dumbbells.

Barbell Presses

● Standing barbell military presses are one of the forever-enduring staples of the weightlifting world. They are a pure test of mind and might against gravity, fear, and spirit. They also work your core muscles and provide a gateway to push presses, allowing you to extend your set even further into the muscle-building zone. There's just something visually distinct about a physique that was built with this exercise. Highly recommended.

● Not all men can perform military presses standing, nor should they on a continuous basis. They are taxing on your lower back. They induce compressive forces on your spine. That's why the seated military press bench was invented.

● Another good military movement is seated with the Smith Machine, especially when you don't have a spotter or want to use partial movements or 21s. Try using both a vertical bench setting as well as a high incline setting. The high incline will help to bring up your upper pecs near the collarbone area.

● The Barbell Press Behind the Neck is an interesting exercise. Although it's highly effective and brings more of the side delt into play, it can also be very dangerous—as in, your weight lifting career is over dangerous. And the danger can rise up suddenly, even if you do everything correctly—fully warmed up, lowering slowly, not too far behind your head, keeping everything in stable alignment. I've seen guys who can regularly do 185lbs in this exercise get seriously injured warming up properly with 95lbs. Why? Because this exercise places your neck/spine and rotator cuffs in precarious positions. One little move of the head, neck extension, etc. can cause discs to herniate, rotator cuffs to tear, etc. Over time, the exercise can wreak havoc on your labrum and rotator cuffs. Do I recommend this exercise? In general, no. But if you must, do it only under certain conditions—as a very occasional movement (use Military presses), typically done with lighter weights and higher reps on a Smith Machine for stability—and only lower the bar to the mid-point behind your head. Otherwise, stick with Military presses—you get pretty much the same benefits with none of the inherent danger.

Dumbbell Presses

- You should master three types of dumbbell shoulder presses: 1) seated on a high incline bench; 2) seated on a vertical bench; and 3) standing (hardest). Using the high incline bench will allow you to hit your upper pec/delt tie-in area, the vertical bench has you pressing in the traditional military style and standing will activate every assistance and stabilization muscle in your body, literally from head to toe (or calves in this case).

- Don't forget about the century old method of one-arm standing dumbbell presses. These helped shape and build the earliest strongmen at the turn of the 20th century, and they can help you pack on additional mass in the 21st century. Try starting with them strict and move to cheating push-presses as you begin to fail. Experiment with a little body English on this one—it's ok.

- Arnold Presses have a slightly greater range of motion since you are able to lower the dumbbells a couple extra inches. This allows your front delts to move through a greater range of motion, which tends to produce more development in the front delt, biceps, and upper chest tie-ins. I'm a big fan of Arnold Presses. I find the most effective strategy is to alternate between Arnold Presses and standard dumbbell presses, using each type of movement for a few weeks before switching to the other.

Front Raises

- You have lots options for front raises, including barbell, dumbbell, cables and plates, as well as range of motion and hand position—palms down or up, hands close or wide—and whether you are standing or seated. Each has advantages and disadvantages.

- Regardless of the type of front raise you perform, make sure you keep your arms straight, your feet flat on the floor and momentum to an absolute minimum. I see too many guys using way too much weight on this exercise, swinging the dumbbells up with their arms bent, their body rocking back and forth or dipping down, while coming up on their toes. That's not a front raise—it's an example of ignorance in the gym. The person willing to put their ego in their back pocket, and concentrate on raising the weight with their anterior deltoid muscle will eventually outperform and build relatively larger front delts than the man with fear.

- Typically, you only need to raise your arms until they are parallel with the floor. This will fully activate the front delts. However, you can raise your arms until they are almost completely overhead—this will bring your traps into play for additional muscle stimulation.

- A close hand position on the barbell will activate some upper inner pec muscle—not a bad thing, especially if you have a weakness there (don't we all?). Similarly, lifting the dumbbell towards the centerline of your chest will produce the same effect.

- Using an underhand grip will work the area where the front delt and upper bicep connect. However, be careful to keep your arms relatively straight here and use a lighter than normal weight. This movement, a past favorite of European weight lifters, can strain biceps tendons if you are not careful.

- Using a neutral grip, with either dumbbells or a rope attached to a cable, provide a similar effect to the underhand option, with less risk to your biceps.

- You can also use a single dumbbell, held with both hands, or an Olympic plate for front raises. Weary souls can even sit sideways on a side lateral machine and perform front raises. All this variety keeps your mind fresh, your workouts interesting and your front delts growing.

- Performing these seated is, of course, the strictest method possible, especially if you keep your back against a military bench pad. Try using a barbell here—although your thighs limit your range of motion, keeping a constant tension on the front delts produces a strong effect.

- An oft-overlooked intensity technique you can use with front raises is 21s. Start with the bottom half of the raise for seven reps, then go to the top half for seven (wow, that gets heavy), and finish with the full range (try to keep body momentum to a minimum). Those things will be on fire. Try these with a cable for even greater intensity.

● Finally, a forgotten movement for front delts is the reverse overhead lateral (dumbbell or cable). This was popular with European bodybuilders several decades ago and really works the front delt, upper pec, bicep tie-in. Just be careful. Use lighter weights and strict form. Hold the dumbbells (or cable handles) at your sides with palms up, and keeping your arms almost straight, lift the weight in an arc to your sides until your hands are overhead. Lower slowly. You should use lighter weights, since this exercise really stresses the upper bicep tendon. Too much weight and you've got a pulled bicep tendon or worse.

Side Laterals

● Side laterals are another in the pantheon of bastardized movements seen in most gyms. I don't know what exercise people think they are doing, but it ain't side laterals. Body rocking fore and aft, arms excessively bent, hands higher than elbows, all on a rearward trajectory akin to a dodo fruitlessly attempting flight. Hopefully, this doesn't describe you.

● Be one of the very few who perform side laterals with dumbbells correctly. A little bend at the elbow is fine, but try to keep your arm as straight as possible and raise the weight directly out to the side. Sitting on a pressing bench with a vertical back will keep you honest most of the time.

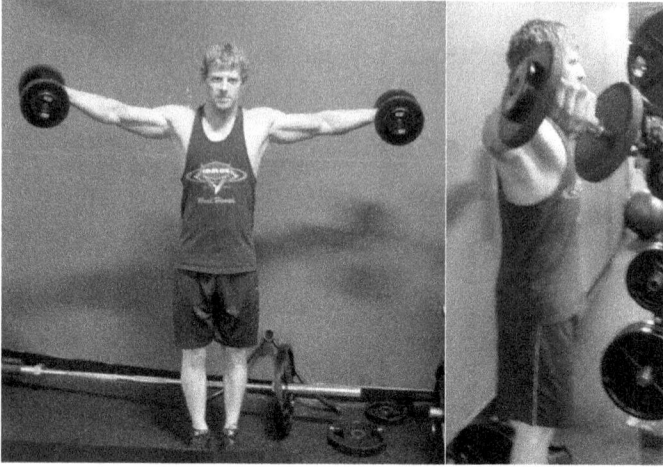

Dumbbell Side Laterals performed strictly

- Here's a trick to help you keep the dumbbells in the correct position— hold them with your pinkie finger against the plates farthest from your body. This will cause them to naturally want to tip forward at the start and help to keep your hand from rotating backward and your elbows up during the movement. A lot of books and instructors will preach about how you should keep your pinkie finger higher than your thumb throughout the movement—just keep them level, not tipped backward (thumb higher than pinkie) and you'll be fine.

- For even stricter form, do these seated, arms locked straight, one arm at a time. Find out just how strong (or weak) your side delts are.

- Every once in awhile, it's a good idea to shock the side delts with some looser form. I've never seen someone build exceptional side delt mass without integrating some planned, controlled loose form with heavy weights in this exercise. Stand up, start with the dumbbells in front of you, lean slightly forward and use some momentum to get the weights up. The key here is to lead with the elbows. Use a weight slightly heavier than you normally use. You can also do this one arm at a time holding onto a support with your free hand.

- Machine side laterals are great for performing 21s. You can also try keeping your arms locked straight as well.

- How high should you lift the weight out to the side? You only need to go to where your elbows are in line with your shoulders—any higher, and you bring your traps into play, which isn't necessarily a bad thing. I recommend lifting your elbows to the height of the top of your head height every third or fourth workout.

- Side laterals and burns go together like peanut butter and chocolate. They often live in isolation, but together they make one hell of an impact. Here's how to make them work for you. At the end of every set, grab a heavier set of dumbbells or select a heavier weight on the stack (about 25-50% heavier) and lift the weight out as high as possible, then hold for a second or two. Do 3-6 burns this way. The key is to perform the burns immediately after normal failure with a weight you cannot get for even a single rep in full range mode. These partial movements will shock your side delts into growth.

- A neglected exercise for your side delts is wide-grip upright rows. Take a grip a little wider than shoulder width and pull the barbell straight up until your arms are in line with your shoulders—no higher. Squeeze the side delt. Use this exercise about once every four side delt sessions.

Rear Laterals

- Rear laterals are one of the few places where I actually recommend a machine over free weights. Why? Because it's much easier to isolate the rear delt head with a rear lateral machine than with dumbbells or cables and it's about the only way you can do them one arm at a time for increased intensity (and find out if one rear delt is stronger than the other). The problem with using dumbbells and cables for rear laterals is threefold—keeping your upper torso parallel to the floor, leading with your elbows (not your hands), and keeping your upper arm motion perpendicular to your shoulders. Typically, even the best of us form gurus tend to lift our torsos upwards as we approach failure. At best, I like to alternate rear laterals between dumbbells and the machine from workout to workout. Free weights are hard to kill.

- Regardless of the type of rear lateral exercise you decide to do, the motion remains the same—it's the exact opposite of the chest fly.

Visualize performing a fly across your back, where you try to touch your elbows together.

- If you are using a rear lateral machine, keep these things in mind: 1) adjust the seat height to an appropriate position—typically, this is where your arms are parallel to the floor; 2) lead with your elbows, not your hands; 3) keep your chest against the pad at all times. Every once in awhile, perform this exercise with your arms locked straight. This exercise is also great for performing 21s as an intensity technique—try it, and you might just discover your rear delt popping out like never before.

- If you are using dumbbells, you may want to try leaning over a preacher bench to stabilize your torso in a position parallel to the floor. This helps to get you in the correct position and keep you from rising up.

- The only type of cable exercise I like for rear laterals is Pulldowns to the Face with a rope attachment. If you've never done this before, here's how you do it. Using a lat pulldown machine, get your thighs locked under the support pad. Lean back slightly, about 20°. Grab the ends of the rope attachment and pull the rope so that each hand ends up beside your ears. Now, hold that position for a second and squeeze your shoulder blades. Slowly return the rope to the starting position, without moving your torso position. This exercise is very effective with higher reps (10-15) and moderate weights, at best. The pull of the rope should affect only your rear delts. If you do this right, you should feel the distinct lactic acid burn in that area.

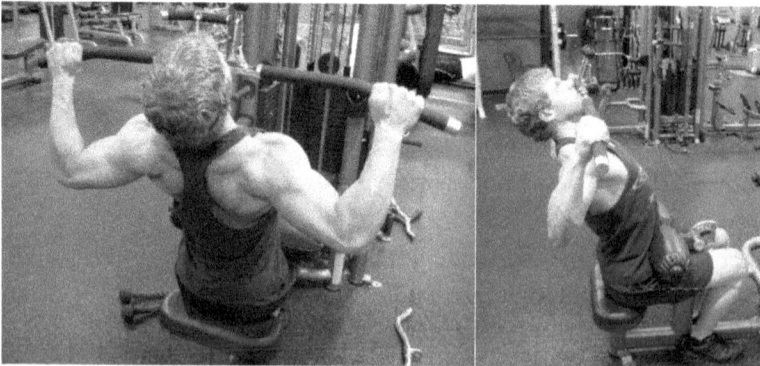

Pulldown to Face—a great exercise to work the rear delts

Traps

Raises the shoulders up.

Key Exercises	Shrugs (Barbell and Dumbbell), Upright Rows
Alternate Exercises	Shrugs and Upright Rows with Cables

General Tips

● There are two key things you'll need to combine in order to build massive traps—very heavy weights and full range of motion. However, you don't necessarily need to do both all the time.

● The bulk of your trap workout should be with weights that you can perform a full range of motion with. Traps really respond well to extreme motion; therefore, you'll need to get those traps shrugged as high as you can and hold them there for a second.

● You'll also need to **incorporate some extremely heavy shrugs into your routine**—weights that are so heavy that you won't be able to get that full range of motion. But what it will do is put an extreme load on your traps—and traps really respond well to extreme weights in shortened ranges. That's why people who do a lot of heavy deadlifts (and no direct trap work) always have large traps.

● Powerlifters will tell you that high pulls will build big traps, and they are right. So will deadlifts. However, for most of us non-powerlifter types, sticking to basic, targeted shrugs and upright rows will build all the traps you ever need or want.

● **Avoid the three common mistakes of shrugs**—bending your arms (check your grip and ego), using a limited range of motion (too much weight), and rotating your shoulders at the top of the movement (stupid).

- Try to **keep your arms straight when shrugging**—otherwise, you are sacrificing some trap activation and bringing those biceps into play. The arms don't need to be locked, just be cognizant of your form when doing these. If you find your arms bending, check the width of your grip on the bar—too narrow of a grip invites bent arms.

- **Don't rotate your shoulders at the top of the shrug**—that's not the purpose of your traps and can cause injury to the rotator cuff and labrum when using heavy weight. Your traps respond best to pulls in a straight plane.

- **Always hold each rep of the shrug at the top of the movement for a second.**

- **Try not to use straps when shrugging.** When you get to the point where your grip is causing you to fail AND you are using extremely heavy weights, then it's ok to strap up.

- Ordinarily, **you shouldn't need to perform any targeted exercises for your neck**. If you are performing heavy deadlifts and shrugs, your neck size should increase accordingly.

Barbell Shrugs

- **You can do barbell shrugs three ways**—standing with the bar either in front or behind you or seated (if you have a cambered bar or Trap Bar). Seated is the strictest, while holding the barbell behind you helps to engage the lower portions of the traps.

- **If you are doing shrugs with the bar behind you, make sure your arms remain straight**—otherwise, you're really performing an upright row behind your back. That's a different movement, with differing results.

- **Try using two barbells, loaded with differing weights, so that you can do drop-sets with shrugs**. This allows you to use a heavy weight for 4-6 reps to increase muscular power and size, and a lighter weight for 10-15 reps for muscular endurance. Best of both worlds and believe me, you'll feel your traps the next day or two.

● To acclimate yourself to holding extremely heavy barbells for shrugs, use the power rack to hold a barbell loaded with a weight that you can only perform for one or two reps. Then, shrug that weight up and hold it there until you reach failure. You can also load on a weight that you can just barely pick up and SLOWLY allow it to stretch your traps in an eccentric (negative) rep. Just be careful with this—concentrate and don't move your head when doing this.

● **Performing shrugs on a Smith Machine is useful for three purposes**—doing strip sets, working your traps when you have a sore lower back, and hitting the lower trapezius muscles near the center of your back. For this latter effect, put the Smith Machine bar at the bottom of the machine, and then set an incline bench at 60° facing backwards right up against the bar. Now, placing your chest against the incline bench, grab a hold of the bar and shrug. Keep your arms completely straight for this. You should feel your mid-back and lower trap area pumping and fatiguing. This is what you want. After a few weeks of this, you should notice your lower traps have more muscle.

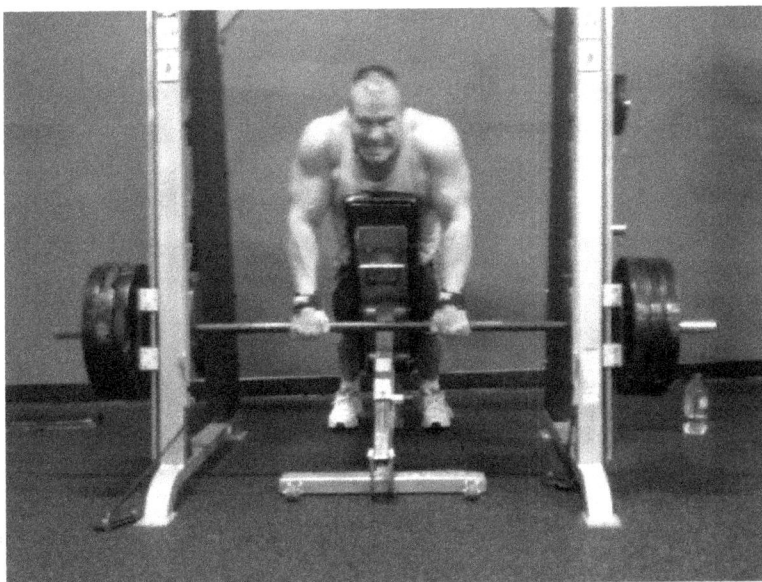

Prone Incline Shrugs on the Smith Machine—all traps, no cheating

● **If your gym has a Trap Bar, you are in luck.** Since this bar places the load at your sides, in line with your body, there is less stress on your lower back. You can even place the bar over a shoulder press bench and do shrugs seated.

Dumbbell Shrugs

● **Dumbbells are the most versatile piece of equipment in any gym. With shrugs, they are no different.** You can perform them standing, seated, or even while moving. You can hold the dumbbells in front of you, to the sides, or behind you. You can even use a reverse grip. You can easily do drop-sets. You can shrug them both at the same time or one at a time. Let's look at a couple techniques to leverage this versatility.

● **Here's an effective technique to end your shrug workout**—grab a set of heavy dumbbells, shrug them up to full contraction and then, either; a) hold them there for as many seconds as you can until your traps give out or, b) walk around the gym like that until your traps start to fatigue. You might get some strange looks if you opt for Plan B, but you just might build some mountains going up to your ears.

● **Dumbbell shrugs and drop-sets are like lovers—they work well together and can produce great results.** It's always good to have options. Try one workout by starting with the heaviest dumbbells (after warming up, of course) and working your way down the rack. For the next workout, try starting at the other end the rack and work your way up. Finally, play both sides and perform drop-set shrugs by alternating heavy and light dumbbells, working your way from each end to the middle.

Cable Shrugs

● **Doing shrugs with cables should not be a part of your normal trap-building routine.** However, occasional use does have one benefit—since you are using a weight stack, you can quickly move the pin to a lighter weight and perform drop-sets. This is always a good way to shock the traps into renewed growth.

Upright Rows

● **Upright rows are a great transitional movement for your front delts, upper pecs, traps and mid-back**—if you do them correctly. Here's how. First, hand width is critical. Place your hands on the bar so that your outstretched thumbs just touch each other. That is how far apart your hands should be (wider positions work more of your side delts). Keep your torso erect, don't lean back, and pull the weight straight up so your hands are even with (or touch) the bottom of your chin. Now, pull your shoulder blades together and squeeze everything hard. Lower the weight UNDER CONTROL to the start position. Some people don't like to pull to the chin, but believe me; this makes a great deal of difference.

● **Since upright rows can be hard on your inner elbow tendons, don't perform this exercise two trap workouts in a row.** Alternate them every other workout.

● You can also do this exercise with dumbbells and cables, but I've found nothing works as well as a barbell for this.

Traps

Biceps

Lifts and curls the arm and turns the wrist up.

Key Exercises	Standing Barbell Curls, Dumbbell Curls, Preacher Curls, Dumbbell Hammer Curls
Alternate Exercises	Incline Dumbbell Curls

General Tips

- **For mass building, your primary biceps exercises should be with barbells and dumbbells.** Leave the cables and machines towards the end of your biceps workout, if at all.

- **The biggest mistake that almost all weight trainers make when working biceps is using a limited range of motion on all types of curls**—especially standing barbell curls and preacher curls, the main workhorses of mass building. Doing that is like putting a restrictor plate on a racecar.

- Other common bicep training mistakes are using too much weight, throwing the weight instead of actually lifting it, using excess body motion and letting the ego drive your workout. They are all inter-related.

- **Stretch your biceps between each set.** I can't say this enough. Try a biceps workout without stretching them and another with stretching. Notice the difference in the pump?

- For overall biceps development, the 'positions of flexion' concept is especially important. Curls can be grouped into four categories, based on where the leverage is most disadvantageous (that's a good thing). You know these types of curls by how hard it is to do the curl at certain points in the movement: at the start (preacher curls), in the mid-range, or sticking point (most curls, especially seated and with cables), and near full contraction (concentration-type curls). I'll look at some strategies for each type below.

- **One of the best intensity techniques to shock the biceps is 21's.** Use them at the beginning of the workout for an intense warm-up, or at the end for a final pump and burn.

- **If all you have access to is a chinning bar, you've got the most basic biceps builder of all.** Before the ancient Greeks invented the pre-cursor to the modern dumbbell (the 'haltere'), man was pulling himself up tree limbs with an underhand grip. Close-grip, underhand chins will build big biceps. Look at any Olympic male gymnast—not a lot of leg mass there, but look at those biceps. What do they do a lot? Pull themselves up holding onto a bar—with an underhand grip.

Barbell Curls

- This is the king of mass builders for the biceps since you are able to use the heaviest weight on them, relative to all other bicep exercises. Perform them both strict and cheating for ultimate results.

- The good way to enforce strict barbell curling is by standing with your back against an upright (use the power rack or something similar).

- You can also perform barbell curls seated from time to time. This mid-range curl is good for breaking through that sticking point that occurs right when the forearms are parallel with the floor. Here, that's your starting position—right at the hardest point. Get stronger on these and your standing barbell curls will improve.

Barbells vs. E-Z Curl Bars

- Let's get this straight right away---the E-Z Curl bar should be renamed the Triceps Bar (it's good for that). It's a sub-optimal curl bar. Why? Because it *reduces* the amount of bicep supination involved. In other words, it reduces the functionality of the biceps. You want your palms completely facing forward when you curl—not turned inward. If you want to turn them inward, then just do hammer curls.

● E-Z Curl bars are still useful—especially when you have a slight wrist or bicep injury. The slight re-positioning of your hands on the bar may allow you to curl without pain. If this is your case, then go for it. But be honest with yourself here—if you can use a barbell instead then you should always opt for the barbell. Unless you want to stick with those same arms you've got.

● E-Z Curl bars are also useful for close-grip barbell curling. Typically, using a narrow grip on a standard barbell is unpleasant on your wrists. The contour of the E-Z curl allows you to perform narrow-grip curls effectively and keep your wrists happy. I would recommend using this type of curl about once every four barbell curling sessions.

● E-Z Curl bars are good for reverse curls—more on this below.

Dumbell Curls

● **Dumbbell curls represent the most complete biceps exercise and the ultimate in versatility.** There are an almost infinite variety of hand position, angles and movement patterns you can assemble each workout to keep your biceps guessing and growing. Unless you have a Roto-bar, it's the only type of free weight curl that allows you to fully supinate your biceps.

● **Try holding the dumbbell handle so your hand is against the inside plate nearest to your body, instead of in the middle of the handle.** As you curl, this will automatically help to turn your wrist outward and supinate the biceps.

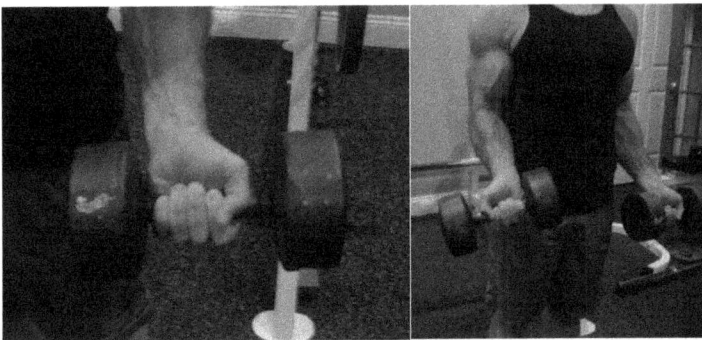

Notice the hand position—against the inside of the dumbbell—this helps turn the wrist out

- A much less used (forgotten?) method of dumbbell curling is to hold one dumbbell with both hands. Hold the dumbbell vertically with your palms under the top plates and curl. You'll find this type of dumbbell curl provides a very different feel and really helps you concentrate of those biceps rolling up and contracting. Work up to heavy weights and you'll see this isn't just for the ladies in the cardio-weight class.

- In the never-ending quest to cheat while performing exercises, most weight trainers tend to dip their body down or shift from side to side in order to get that weight up on a curl. Don't do that. If you see yourself doing this, sit down in a narrow space and curl.

- If you perform your dumbbell curls while lying on a flat bench (a seemingly lost form of curls), then be careful with the upper bicep attachment into your shoulder girdle. You don't want an injury in that area. Always use lighter weights and higher reps if performing this form of curl. While danger lurks (not unusual in any type of exercise), it's a useful alternative for an occasional shock to the biceps—they aren't expecting a curl from this position.

- Everybody likes a two-for-one deal. Zottman curls give you that. For those unfamiliar with this curl of yesteryear, you start by performing a regular dumbbell curl. After squeezing your biceps hard at the top, turn your wrist down and lower the dumbbell slowly under control. What you are doing is performing the negative of a reverse curl. So, Zottman's give you a regular dumbbell curl and part of a reverse curl in one movement— a veritable bargain for your biceps. If you want to ratchet up the intensity on this exercise, perform it on the preacher bench.

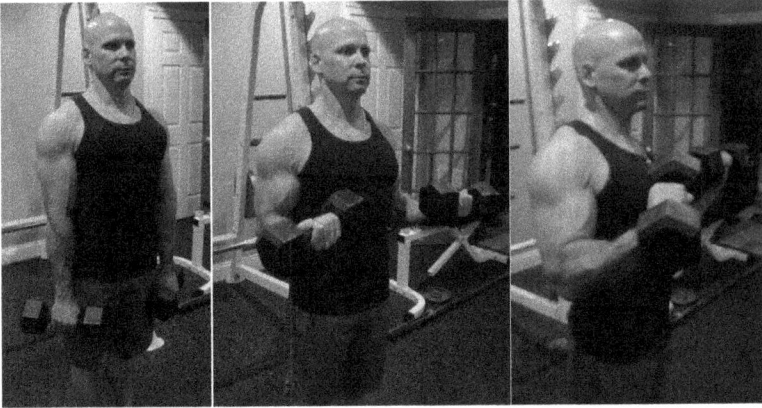

The Zottman Curl—regular curl on the way up, reverse curl on the way down

Hammer Curls

- **Regular use of hammer curls does two things: makes your arms appear wider (thicker) when viewed from the front and builds bigger forearms.** That's because curling a weight with a neutral, thumbs-up grip shifts most of the stress to the brachialis and brachioradialus muscles which, when developed, make the forearm extensor muscles bigger and push the biceps muscle up and out, since the brachialis lies under the biceps.

- **You can do hammer curls two ways**: by bringing the dumbbell across the front of your body or by using the more traditional method of bringing it straight forward like a normal dumbbell curl. What's the difference? Not much, but you will probably be able to use more weight with the across your body approach, due to pure physics (a weight held farther from your body is harder to lift). Most people tend to cheat with this approach, and that's ok here. Just think of it this way—today, do you want to stress your biceps/forearms with a little more weight, but looser form, or go slightly lighter but strict? Can't decide? Try alternating each approach from workout to workout. Think of it as Dollar Cost Averaging for the arms.

- **For the ultimate in strict hammer curling, combine hammer curls with spider curls to get hammer spider curls.** Absolutely no cheating there. If you don't have a dedicated spider curl bench (and what gym does?), you can turn the opposite way on the preacher bench and hang your arm straight down the backside.

- **If you have access to a triceps bar with the neutral hand position grips, that's a great bar to use for hammer curls.** It tends to keep the exercise very strict. For an even stricter application of hammer curls with this bar, combine it with preacher or spider curls. This variation is always useful if you need to get your form back in check.

Preacher Curls

- **The preacher bench is the place to answer most of your prayers for bigger biceps.** What God didn't provide you, you can create yourself here. This bench can not only make biceps bigger, but also accentuates thickness, lower bicep mass and peak, depending on hand position, bench use, and proper form. The variety of things you can do here is almost endless: use dumbbells, cable or barbell, regular, reverse, hammer and concentration curls, use partials and burns, etc. Let your imagination reign.

- Larry Scott stated that the pot of gold on the preacher curls lies at the bottom of the curl, where you need to fully stretch the biceps before initiating the curl. How true. However, where there is reward, there is usually risk. In this case, peril waits if you lower the weight too quickly to the fully stretched position--hyperextension of the elbow, tendons and bicep muscle can occur. Always lower the weight slowly, under control on this exercise.

- **The key to preacher curls is two-fold**—full extension at the bottom AND a strict fight through the early stage of the curl with absolutely no body movement for cheating purposes.

- **There are two ways to preacher curl—standing or sitting—and each has its own positional trick to maximize the effectiveness.** If standing, dig your armpits into the pad, letting your entire body weight rest on the pad, while your legs are either completely forward under the pad or straight out behind you. Either way, don't use your legs to support your weight. Only use them for balance purposes, if at all. If sitting, adjust the seat height so that your armpits are firmly into the pad, but not so low that you risk hyperextension when your arms are fully extended. If unsure, err on the side of a higher seat height setting.

● **Preacher curls can be hard on the elbows and tendons.** It's a good idea to use preacher curls every other biceps workout so the elbows and tendons can remain healthy.

● **Never perform preacher curls first in the bicep workout.** You really need to warm up the biceps, elbow and tendons in that area by performing another type of curl first.

Reverse Curls

● **Reverse curls with a barbell are like the bicep exercise that time forgot.** Weight lifters of the 1950s always did this exercise, and no surprise, they all seemed to have huge forearms and thick biceps. Weight trainers of today don't typically perform reverse curls, let alone reverse curls with a barbell. Those that do, migrate toward the E-Z Curl bar for this exercise, since it does take a lot of the stress off the wrist—but also reduces the effectiveness of the exercise. Try varying hand widths on the bar and find a width that allows your wrists to co-exist peacefully with this exercise. You will be surprised at the results.

● A big problem with reverse curls, regardless of the bar used, is that we tend to like cheating the weight up on this type of curl, maybe more so than any other variation. One remedy is to perform reverse curls using the preacher bench.

Concentration Curls

● **Concentration-type curls have a bad name.** You should be concentrating on all types of curls, not just these peak-contraction type of curls. What makes these types of curls different is that they place the biceps under intense load near the fully contracted position of the curl. Examples of this type of curl include seated or standing dumbbell concentration curls, spider curls (barbell or dumbbell), lying overhead cable curls, and cable crossover curls.

● While many trainees like to perform concentration curls seated with a dumbbell, their upper arm resting against their thigh, I prefer several alternative forms which I think are superior for inducing stress—standing with your arm hanging straight down (don't let that upper arm move from vertical), standing using a cable (same warning), standing concentration curls with the cable crossover, and spider curls.

● **Spider curls are probably the most intense form of concentration curl—if you do them strictly.** Since most gyms don't have a spider curl bench, use the vertical side of the preacher curl bench. Grab a barbell or dumbbell and lean over the vertical edge of the bench, letting your upper arm hang straight down. Now keep it there throughout the entire exercise. Failure to do so will turn this from an exceptional peak builder to a poor man's bicep curl. More than anything else, the key here is form and squeezing the biceps at the top of the curl. The weight is secondary. Once you've squeezed as hard as you can, squeeze a little harder.

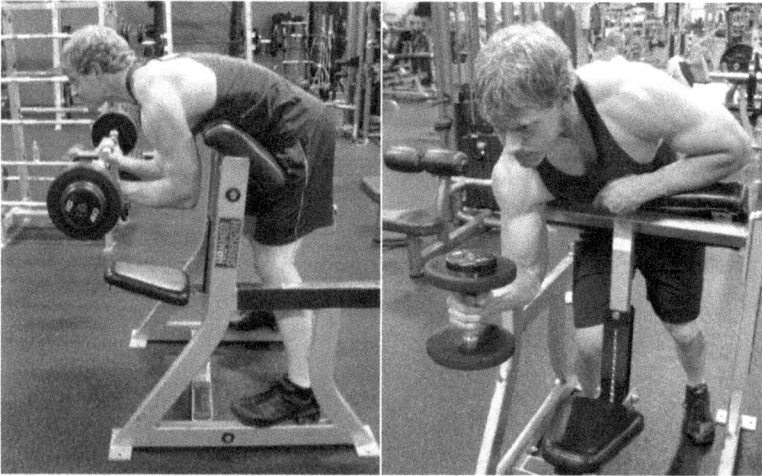

Use the reverse side of the Preacher Curl bench for Spider Curls—keep those upper arms vertical

● Standing concentration curls using the cable crossover cables are another excellent exercise that mimics the bodybuilder's front double biceps pose.

When to Use Cable Curls

● Cable curls are useful, since they provide a uniform tension during the entire range of the curl, unlike free weight curls, which provide most of the tension during the first half of the curl.

Using an Arm Blaster

● There is a reason that Arm Blaster type devices have been around for four decades—they work. They work because they significantly reduce the amount of cheating that most weight trainers use when working biceps. Sure, you'll see guys using an Arm Blaster swinging their body forward and back, but their upper arms remain in line with their torso—a vast improvement over the complete abandonment of proper form which has become ritual.

● **To get the most out of the Arm Blaster, keep your upper body from swinging forward and back during most of your set.** Only for the last rep or two should you employ a little body English to get the weight past the sticking point. Make sure to start each rep with your arms hanging completely straight at full extension—you won't believe how much harder and effective it makes the exercise. The pump you get will be much greater this way.

● **Use of the Arm Blaster brings one hidden danger**—since the device restricts backward movement of your upper arms, you need to be especially careful when lowering the weight. I said 'lowering'—not 'dropping'. If your typical form entails heaving up the heaviest barbell/dumbbell you can, then quickly dropping it back down, to heave it up again, you are in for a big injury surprise. The backwards restriction, coupled with any dropping to a full extension can easily result in hyperextension of the biceps, at that, my friend is a painful companion to carry around with you for months. Bicep hyperextensions are notoriously slow to heal, since your biceps are involved with so much you do in daily life. You have been warned. Form is essential for longevity here.

● Don't forget—besides barbell and dumbbell curls, the Arm Blaster is great for hammer, reverse and Zottman curls.

- **Don't rely on the Arm Blaster for your biceps workouts.** Think about it—it's a crutch for those who don't/can't seem to be able to use proper curling form. I think the best use of it is as an occasional reminder or reinforcement mechanism when you think your form needs a kick back into place.

- If you don't have an Arm Blaster, don't worry. You can perform your curls while standing against an upright, such as a power rack.

Triceps

Straightens the arm and turns the wrist down.

Key Exercises	Close-Grip Bench Press, Dips, Pushdowns, Barbell Extensions (Lying/Seated)
Alternate Exercises	Dumbbell Extensions, Kickbacks

General Tips

- **Two-thirds of your upper arm mass is triceps.** The long head of the triceps is the largest triceps muscle. Think about that.

- **Since the primary purpose of the triceps is to straighten the arms, all triceps work boils down to dips, presses, pushdowns and extensions.** However, those four types of movements open an almost limitless world of possibilities.

- **For pure mass building, there is nothing like close-grip bench presses and dips.** Both are multi-joint movements. Surprise. Bigger and stronger triceps produced through close-grip benches and dips produce stronger bench presses and bigger pecs. If you find someone that has big triceps but a small chest, you found someone who probably uses mostly single joint triceps movements in lieu of presses/dips. You also found someone who is asymmetrical.

- **When doing any type of triceps exercise, don't accelerate your arms into a straightened position**—this will cause all kinds of elbow issues as you age. You want to decelerate as you reach full contraction, and then squeeze all hell out of your triceps.

- **Triceps love negatives.** You can use this intensity technique on presses and dips. I wouldn't suggest using it with pushdowns or extensions.

- Always perform your biceps workout (or a biceps exercise, if supersetting between bis/tris) before triceps. This will warm up your elbows, tendons and triceps and provide a nice cushion when performing your triceps exercises. Another good tactic is to alternate bicep and triceps exercises—this tends to keep both muscles full of blood.

- **Stretch your triceps between each set.** The best way to stretch the triceps is by holding a rolled up towel in your hand, extend your arm overhead, lower your hand behind your head, have your workout partner add resistance by pulling on the other end of the towel, while you attempt to perform an extension. You should feel the triceps stretch all the way into your rear delt area. If you don't have a towel or a partner, hold onto an upright with your hand and lean into it while allowing your triceps to fully stretch. Hold the stretch for 5-10 seconds.

Dips

- **Dips are the king of triceps mass builders.** Look at the size of any male Olympic gymnast's triceps and you'll see the results of hundreds of thousands of dips.

- The best apparatus for this movement is dedicated thick-handled dipping bars, which are angled to allow a range of widths. Most gyms don't have these (if yours does, thank the weightlifting gods). You'll have to make do with some dipping handles attached a power rack, chin station, etc. You can use a bench as a last resort.

- Since dips can be used to work either triceps or chest (or both at once, although not optimally), it's important to get the correct form down. You want to keep your torso as vertical as possible—try not to lean forward too much. The more you lean forward, the more you bring the chest into play (essentially performing a decline or flat bench press movement). We want to hit the triceps as hard as possible here, so stay upright.

- **Typically, your hand width should be at shoulder width or slightly less**, but feel free to try various widths and note the effect.

- **Lower yourself until your upper arms are parallel with the floor.** Below parallel and you bring more chest and shoulders into play (and it can be hard on your shoulders depending on your flexibility, joint strength, etc.). Above parallel and you are doing partial reps.

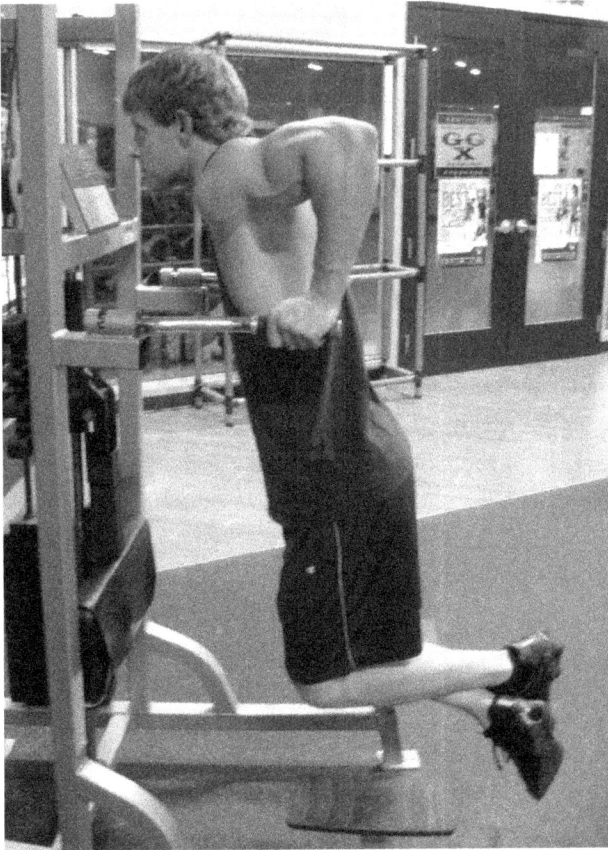

● Press yourself up (staying upright) until you reach lockout or just before lock-out—your choice. Locking out allows you to really squeeze the triceps hard and etch in detail, while not locking out keeps continuous tension on the triceps and makes the movement harder. Alternating both methods is a good choice.

● **Using a dipping belt really allows you to pack on the muscle here.** Even if you can't do a full rep with some really heavy plates strapped on, you can perform beneficial partials.

Close-Grip Presses

● **If Dips are the king of triceps mass builders, then close-grip presses are next in line to the throne.** You can do this multi-joint movement on incline, flat and decline benches. While the flat version is most common, the incline version is great for building upper/inner pecs, as well as triceps. The decline version introduces a shorter range of motion, allowing you to use heavier weights. However, unless you have a weakness with your lower/inner pecs (probably not), stick with the flat and incline varieties. There are better methods for increasing close-grip pressing power, detailed below.

● Common mistakes in this exercise include incorrect hand spacing, bouncing the bar off the chest, lowering the bar too low, arching the back, and not keeping a stable base. Your hands should be 12-14" apart. If you were taught to keep your hands closer, I bet you have some sore wrists at higher weights. Don't worry, even at 14" apart, your triceps will be doing most of the work and not your chest—and your wrists will appreciate it. The bar should be lowered to mid-chest (nipple area) or slightly higher. Keep your feet flat on the floor. Don't lift your heels—this tends to assist in excessive back arching—you don't want that, since the stress will start to shift to your front delts. If you have trouble keeping your back flat on the bench, try putting your feet up on the bench.

● You can press the weight one of two ways—to full lockout or almost to lockout. I prefer almost to lockout, since none of the stress is taken off the triceps, giving you a continuous tension effect.

● **Partial reps are a great way to increase your strength on this exercise.** Use a power rack or the Smith Machine for this. If you use a power rack, you can use the same three-position technique described in the Chest section for barbell presses.

● **If you are use a Smith Machine, try doing 21s or drop-sets**. You won't have to worry about balancing the weight as you take your triceps to new levels of muscular fatigue.

Pushdowns

● **The only cable-based movement you need for triceps is pushdowns.** There is a continuum of form on this exercise—from absolutely strict (elbows in, no leaning) to power pushdowns (elbows out, leaning into weight), with most people using something in between. The two extremes are useful for carving in detail and adding hunks of mass. Just be cognizant of which type you need to perform based on your goals.

- Any time that you have a cable attached to a stack of weight, you have an opportunity for drop-sets and 21s. For pushdowns, this is no different.

- There are numerous variations of pushdowns based on hand position (palms down or up, neutral grip), type of attachment (V-bar, straight, angular, rope), hand width (narrow, shoulder-width, wide), and whether you are performing them one arm at a time or with both. Master all these variations and you will be rewarded with shapely and detailed triceps, given the mass you build with dips and presses.

- One-arm pushdowns will help you expose which arm's triceps muscles are stronger/weaker. Use this knowledge to your advantage and correct the imbalance.

- A common mistake when using a rope attachment for pushdowns is turning your wrists outward at the bottom of the movement. What you want to do is set a linear path from start to finish, where you start with your hands close, but finish with them far apart. Don't forget to hold that contraction.

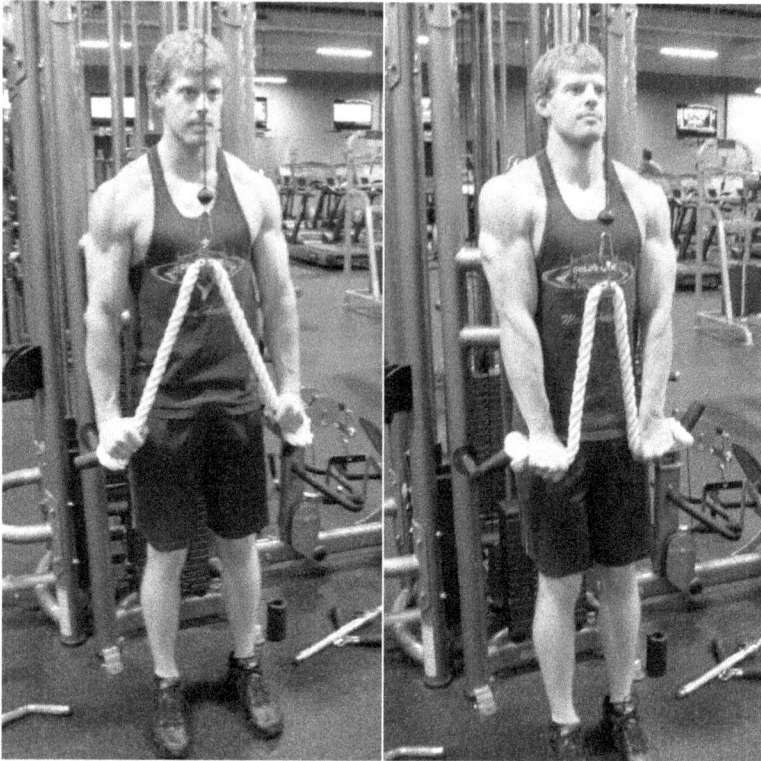

Correct (left) and incorrect (right) form with the Rope Pushdown

A World of Extensions

● There is a seemingly endless variety of triceps extension movements you can perform. Most of these variations can be classified by equipment—barbell, dumbbell or cable, position (standing, seated, lying), angle of movement, and whether you are using one arm or both at the same time. However, there is one gem of knowledge hiding in all these options lying before you—the long head of the triceps is the key to massive upper arm size and certain types of extensions can help you build it.

● **The long head of the triceps makes up about 50% of your total upper arm size.** Read that again. So, shouldn't you concentrate on building up that sucker as much as you can? Yes, Virginia, you should. A quick anatomy lesson is useful here. The long head of the triceps runs from the back of your shoulder to your elbow. Important point—it attaches to the back of your shoulder. Therefore, in order to use a full range of motion with this muscle, from complete stretch to contraction, requires that your elbow be beside your head. That means overhead extensions. You can do them standing, sitting, with a barbell, dumbbells or a cable, but you must keep your elbows beside your head—and you must do them consistently with heavy weight. Use a barbell for the quickest results.

● **Keep in mind that barbell extensions can be hard on your elbows and tendons.** For this reason, try to perform this movement every other workout, at most. You have to balance the time attainment of your goals with longevity. In addition, just because you are doing barbell extensions doesn't mean you shouldn't adjust your hand width from workout to workout.

● Here's a great variation of 21s for lying barbell extensions ("skull crushers")—lower the bar behind your head for the first seven reps, to your forehead for the next seven, and to your chin for the final seven. This will adjust the range of motion and angle of attach through the 21 reps.

● If you are doing a dumbbell extension (two hands, one dumbbell) behind your head, be careful not to go too low—don't touch the base of your neck. This movement introduces a similar shoulder position as presses behind the neck and can put your upper spine in a precarious position if your elbows flare out.

● One-arm, overhead dumbbell extensions are a popular movement, especially with women who want to get rid of that flabby underarm (by working the long head, of course). Just make sure you keep your elbow pointed straight up to the ceiling—if your elbow starts to drift off toward your shoulder, you are cheating. This is ok for the last rep or two—just don't make that form part of your normal routine.

● **When performing a standing or kneeling cable extension to build up the long head, try to keep your elbows higher than your head** (as described above). The best variation of this movement is kneeling, with your elbows supported on a bench and your head slightly below the height of the bench. Try using a rope—this will really allow you to stretch your triceps. You should feel a pump and burn all the way to the back of your shoulder if you are doing this correctly.

- **Lying dumbbell extensions are a good alternative to a barbell.** They will allow you to lower the bells beside your head for a greater stretch and range of motion.

- Keep in mind that when you are deciding to do extensions either standing/seated or lying flat or on a decline, you shorten the range of motion as you move from standing/seated to decline. Sometimes, due to injury, a shortened range of motion can keep you working this exercise without pain.

- **Seated barbell extensions (use an E-Z Curl Bar if you have wrist issues) are one of the best long-head builders**, so make sure you spend a lot of time with these. Clean the weight from the floor to your shoulders, sit down, and press the weight overhead to start. Keep your elbows in, lower the weight, and go for a full stretch. The range of motion you can get here is more important than the weight. Don't sacrifice weight for form on this exercise or you'll never get the full benefit. Use two dumbbells for an occasional change from the barbell.

- **Standing barbell extensions are the old school mass builder for the long head.** Everybody these days likes to sit when standing is often a better alternative. Take the harder route and do them standing. This will allow you to use slightly more weight, body momentum and some cheating to really pack on the mass. Just balance this form with the stricter seated variety.

Kickbacks

- I'm not a big fan of kickbacks in any form, since you are not going to add much muscle with this exercise. You can get all the triceps development you need from the other exercises in this section. However, if you are going to do them as an occasional break from your regular work, at least do them correctly.

- The most common mistakes are using too much weight, not keeping your arm at the best angle (related to using too much weight), and not contracting at the top of the movement. Here's what you want to do—you upper arm should be locked at the side of your torso, parallel to the floor (not pointing downward), and you should only move at the elbow joint until you completely lock out the weight and hold it in the contracted position for a second.

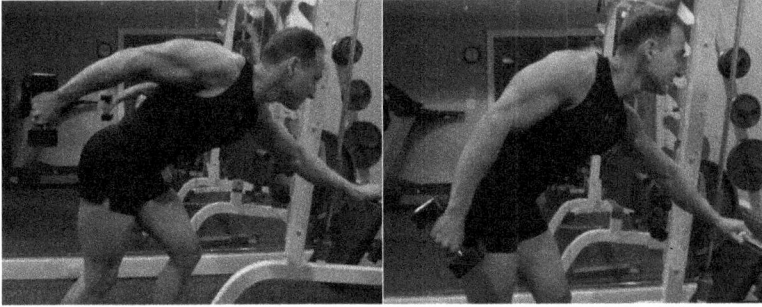

Correct (left) and incorrect (right) kickback form—keep the upper arm parallel to the floor

● Try turning your palm up at contraction—this will intensify the contraction.

The Forgotten Ones

● Ever seen someone do a Pullover & Press for their triceps? Probably not. That's too bad, since this multi-joint exercise, popular decades ago, built some great triceps, as well as front delts, pecs, and serratus muscles. Try it, show your friends, and build a nice flowing physique. Grab a barbell, lie back on a bench, and press the weight up. Now, lower the weight to your chest, then move the bar, under control, until it moves up to your head, just over your face, then lower it down behind your head. Reverse the movement. Pull the bar up and over your torso (ala pullovers) and then press it up like a standard bench press. That's one rep. Try sets of 6-8 reps with ever increasing weights and watch how your triceps and entire upper torso start to pump up like a Macy's Thanksgiving Day float. Keep this up and you might win a prize.

● I'm not sure why, but somewhere along the way, when guys starting picking up weights, they stopped doing push-ups. Big mistake. The ladies don't seem to be as stupid about this. Even though push-ups limit you to your body weight (unless you take some creative measures), they are still excellent for warming up or doing drop-sets after a pressing movement. For your triceps, just keep your hands closer than shoulder width when you do them.

Forearms

Curls the palm up and down.

Key Exercises	Forearm Curls (Barbell and Dumbbell), Reverse Forearm Curls (Barbell and Dumbbell)
Alternate Exercises	Forearm Curls and Reverse Curls with Cables

General Tips

- **The best method to develop strong, muscular forearms is probably to just hold onto some really heavy weights.** A great way to do this while building a strong back is to perform deadlifts with no straps. Another good candidate is heavy shrugs without straps. In fact, try performing all of your exercises without straps. If you typically use straps, especially on exercises such as pull-downs and rows, your forearms should be pretty sore the next day. If you have trouble holding a pen or pencil, you did real good. Just remember, forearms are tough suckers, so don't expect that level of soreness to continue.

- Another technique to bring up weak forearms indirectly is to perform a few sets of just holding onto an extremely heavy barbell (something that's around your 1RM for barbell shrugs) in a power rack at the end of every workout. You should be doing this 3-5 times per week—every time you workout. Hold the barbell until your grip gives out. While holding, squeeze your forearms as hard as you can. Do this three times, and then you're ready to hit the showers.

- If you weren't blessed with good forearm genetics, have used the no-strap philosophy described above, and still have lackluster forearms, you'll need to incorporate some direct forearm work into your arm routine. Start treating forearm work with as much emphasis as you place on any other body part.

● There's really only two types of direct forearm work you can do—wrist curls and reverse wrist curls. However, there are many variations and techniques you can employ to make the most of this duo.

● **The key to both wrist curls and reverse wrist curls is the height of your hips in relation to your forearms**. What? Typically, when you perform wrist curls—with a barbell, dumbbells, whatever—you sit on a bench with your forearms resting on the top of your thighs as you bend forward and use your wrists to curl. That's not a very productive position in terms of leverage, power, range of motion, etc. Most benches are designed for performing just about every type of upper body exercise effectively, except forearms. What you need is a bench that's high enough that you can rest just your forearms on it, and kneel, sit or stand so that your hips are lower than your forearms resting on that bench. You need a forearm curl bench. You're going to have to improvise one. The best methods I've found are to either rest your forearms on the top of the preacher curl bench or put a couple 45lb plates under a regular bench to set it higher off the floor, then sit on the floor with your forearms on the bench. With either method, your forearms should be higher than your hips. That's the whole key—setting up your wrist curl positioning optimally. Do this and all other variations of wrist curls (behind the back, at the sides with dumbbells, etc.) become second-rate.

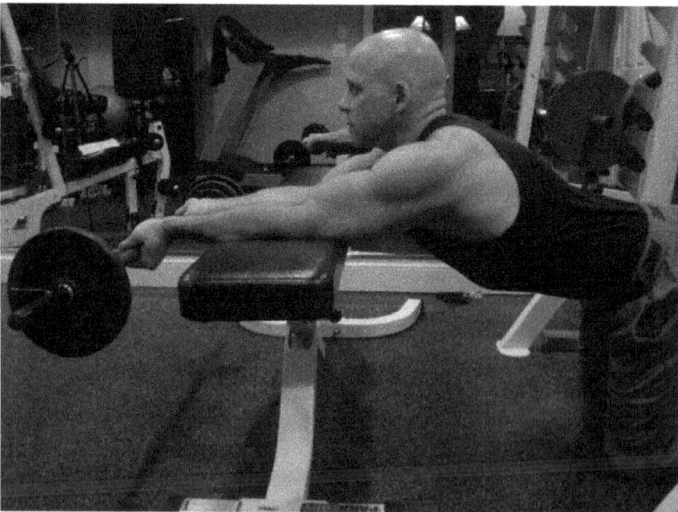

Effective forearm curls—hips lower than forearms, full stretch

- You'll find that you can't use anywhere near the same amount of weight on reverse wrist curls versus wrist curls. That's normal. I've found that the best exercise to develop the brachioradialus and the forearm extensors (the top of your forearm) is the barbell reverse curl. Note that I said 'barbell' reverse curl—don't use an E-Z curl bar if you want optimal development here. You need that wrist turned down.

- A final thought to keep in mind—any weight that you can wrist curl, you can bicep curl. Think about that. So, if you increase the amount you can wrist curl…☺

Forearms

Quads

Extends and straightens the leg.

Key Exercises	Squats, Front Squats, Hack Squats, Leg Extensions, Leg Presses
Alternate Exercises	Smith Machine Squats, Box Squats, Box Front Squats, Single Leg Press

General Tips

- The three big rules for keeping your knees healthy over time are: 1) warm-up with leg extensions; 2) use proper form, and 3) don't bounce at the bottom of squats.

- **There is just no way around this—if you want exceptional legs, you must squat.** You can leg press all you want, but if you don't squat, you'll never get the level of development that squats bring. In fact, you can visually identify those that squat and those that don't. Below, I'll talk about specific techniques and tips you can use for a variety of types of squats.

- **Most quad exercises are overrated or a waste of time, including lunges and adductor machines.** Try to stick with the big boys—squats and leg presses. If you have lower back or knee problems, then leg presses and extensions are your best bet.

- **It's a good idea to start with leg extensions to warm up the knee joints and pre-fatigue the quads.** That way, you won't have to go quite as heavy on the squats. Your lower back will get less stress applied and this simple warm-up will keep your knees healthy for decades.

- **Every day after a quad workout should be a rest day.** An intense quad workout has a systemic effect on the entire body—it will deplete all your energy reserves.

- Typically, your glutes will develop in conjunction with your quads and lower back, due to all the heavy squats and deadlifts you are performing (you are performing them, aren't you?).

- If you need extra work to bring up your glute size or shape, you can perform wide-stance (duck) squats and reverse lunges.

Leg Extensions

- **There are two purposes for leg extensions**—to get your knees warmed up for the squats and presses to follow, and to carve in separation and detail into your quads. After all, you do want to show the world that quads are made of four separate muscles, don't you? To get the most out of this exercise, you need to do a couple things.

- Adjust the backrest on the machine so that just the lower part of your quads with your knees clears the seat. You don't want too much quad hanging over, but you also don't want the back of your lower leg smack up against the pad either. Find the right adjustment setting and use that from now on. It's all about leverage, effectiveness, and healthy knees.

- Two points of execution are important—use a full range with a strong contraction at the top, and don't let your rear end come up off the seat, especially as you work with heavier weight. Coming up off the seat effectively cuts down your range of motion and the effectiveness of the exercise. Remember; always work to make things harder, not easier. The hard path is the path to success in weight lifting.

- For your last rep, try holding the peak contraction for as long as you can—it makes a big difference over time.

- Try varying how close your thighs are when seated. Keep them together for a set or workout, then next time put them as far apart as the machine will allow. You should notice that wide equals more inner quad development, while a close stance produces more stress on the outer quad. A good strategy is rotate between close, normal, and wide across three workout sessions, then repeat. You should be noticing a theme by now with this three-position stuff.

- Every fourth workout on this exercise, try doing it one leg at a time. This will allow you to monitor for subtle degrees of weakness between quads, something not so easily determined with squats.

- **For the ultimate in leg extension intensity, try performing 21s**—first seven reps the beginning half of the extension, next seven the top half, and final seven the whole range of motion. Hold at the last rep, and then excuse yourself to the rest room. Didn't think you could ever feel queasy after a set of leg extensions, did you?

Squats

- In this section, I'll talk about the emperor of squats—the traditional back squat. Following sections will give you some insights regarding other types of squats—listed in order of effectiveness.

- **The type of footwear you use for squats is important.** Try to use shoes that have a wide, flat base-something like a basketball court shoe. Some like combat boots for this purpose (squats do present a war of sorts—with both mind and body). Of course, actual weight lifting shoes are best. You may also want to try taking your shoes off and squatting in just your socks. There's nothing like your feet against the Earth for the sheer brutality of the lift.

- **Basically, you can do squats with the bar two places on your back**—the traditional powerlifting method where the bar is lower down your upper back or the high-bar method, where the bar sits on the top of your traps. I prefer the high-bar method, since I think it helps to instill more of an upright torso—and you aren't a powerlifter. Whatever method you prefer, make sure your torso does not bend forward excessively. Your lower back won't like that.

- Where to look, where to look? Some squatting advocates say to look slightly up when squatting; others say look straight ahead, etc. Seems there are as many opinions on this as compass positions. Since most squat racks are in front of a mirror, stare at the floor in the mirror at a point about 10 feet forward (this should be slightly down from the straight-ahead option)—that one stares into infinity—we want you grounded.

● **Please, dear lord, if you are going to squat, then actually perform a squat—not a curtsy.** Don't flirt with the squat—get your ass down into the basement and see if you have what it takes to actually drive a pile of weight against the full gravitational force of the Earth. If you actually take the time to learn the squat correctly with light weight—down to parallel, no excessive forward lean, no rounding of the back—you will eventually be able to squat more than most humans could ever imagine. Take the time to burn that motion into your psyche. In this case, the tortoise really does win the race. Oh, and guys that do only half squats end up with legs shaped like a carrot—big at the top, narrowing down to pencil-like size at the knees. I don't have to tell you that looks bad.

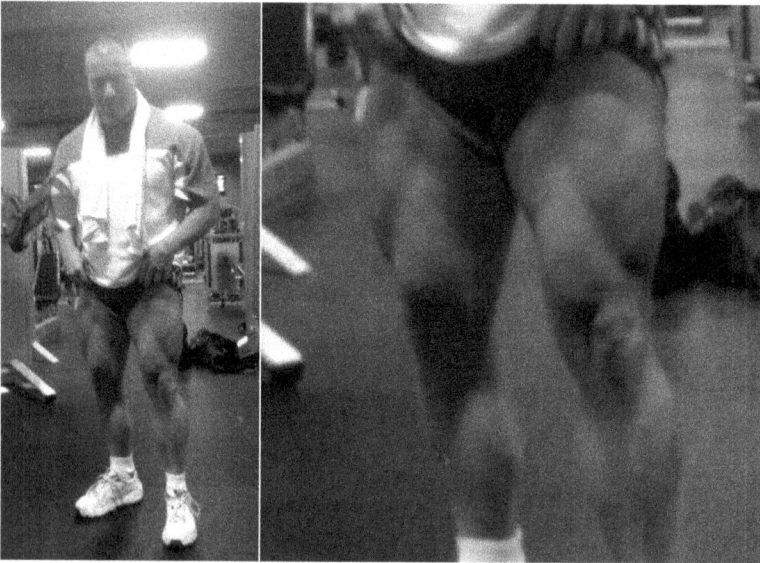

Yes, the author has quads

● **Have someone you trust (and that's honest with you) evaluate your form on squats occasionally.** This will tend to catch any minor problems with form and allow you to make slight adjustments. You don't want bad habits to form—and they can form, even after years of experience. This is good advice for just about any exercise.

● **When squatting, it's often good to alternate between foot stance widths**: narrow (slightly less than shoulder width), standard (shoulder width or slightly wider) and wide (much wider than shoulder width—also like a duck squat). To gauge the proper widths, it's helpful to place two 25lb. plates on the floor inside of the squat rack. For the narrow stance, place the outer sides of your feet/shoes against the side of the plates. The plates act as a guide so that you get a consistent width of stance each time.

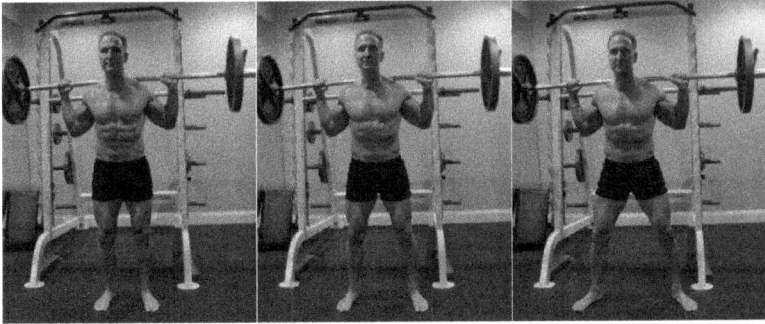

Squats with narrow, normal, and wide stances. You are only as strong as your weakest stance.

● **Learn to love the bottom—of the squat movement that is.** Most people can't wait to get down then back up in the squat. The real gold in a squatting movement starts with that just below parallel position. Yes, contrary to what your girlfriend or wife says, an inch or two really does matter. So, don't cheat yourself and stop before you get to that bottom position. Drop the weight if you have to—don't worry, if you learn to go this low, then your quads will reward you in the end. Try teaching yourself to hold the bottom position for a second before pushing the weight back up.

● **Using a partial range of motion on squats is useful for several reasons**—first, it helps you to mentally handle some really heavy weight, a weight you can't currently use with full range. Once you get your mind wrapped around the fact that you have 500lbs on your back and you can control it, things start to fall into place for that next phase of your squatting career. Second, it helps to build explosive power in the hips and put some additional mass on the upper portions of your quads. Finally, doing squats with only the bottom half of the movement increases overall squatting strength and power. Do these partial movements in a power-rack.

- **When squatting, if you find your knees moving inward, that means that you have weak adductor muscles.** You have to remember that you are only as strong as your weakest link. In this case, you are weakest when performing wide stance squats. Get your strength up in wide stance squats (do more of them) and your knees will stop moving inward. This is why we advocate performing squats with varied foot widths—and, your quads will achieve better overall shape.

- **Every fourth quad workout should be a non-squat workout.** This helps the back recuperate from the spinal compression of the previous weeks and provides a mental break.

- **Every couple of months is a good time to perform 10 sets of 10 reps in the standard squat.** This really puts the quads through an intense workout that also incorporates volume training. Quads like volume.

- Women who squat consistently will develop legs and glutes that can't be duplicated with other movements.

Front Squats

- **Front squats are the movement that nobody wants to do, but boy, do they make a difference.** They're tough, as well as one of the harder athletic movements to perform with weights. Additionally, they will show you and everyone else just how much quad power you really have. Regular performance of front squats will be rewarded with sizeable and shapely quads—quads which typically display amazing outer sweep. No other exercise can produce this effect.

- You can't cheat on this exercise—since your upper torso needs to remain pretty much vertical, cheating will cause the bar to fall forward, ending the set. Due to this vertical alignment, front squats are much easier on your lower back, since your lower back does very little with this movement. It's pretty much all quads, baby.

- **The trick to perfecting your form on this exercise is to constantly force your elbows to stay up.** This will keep your torso erect and the stress off your lower back and on your quads where it belongs.

Hack Squats

- **Hack squats are a great outer quad sweep builder and they help thicken your quads down near the knee** (no more carrot legs), but you have to do them correctly. This means a full range of motion—you need to go to where your quads and your lower legs have slightly less than a 90° angle—in other words, the same depth you are using with your squats and leg presses. Also, don't come all the way up on each rep—keep constant tension on the quads—this, coupled with full range, magnifies the effectiveness of this exercise.

- **Hack squats can also be hard on your knees**—that's why I recommend doing them every other leg workout, at most. Over time, this will reduce the amount of accumulated stress placed on your knees. Make sure you place your feet appropriately on the platform—typically, this will be towards the top of the platform. Placing your feet low on the platform increases the stress on your knees.

- Make sure you alter the width of your stance on the platform (just like on the leg press)—a good strategy is to alternate between normal, narrow, and wide stances for complete development.

Smith Machine Squats

- **Performing squats on the Smith Machine is a good alternative if you want to go heavy and don't have a spotter or power rack available.** They can also be good if you have a sore lower back and need to stabilize and/or limit your range of motion somewhat. They're also useful for performing duck squats—squats with a very wide stance, or squats with your feet farther forward of your body for occasional variation.

- **Make sure you position your feet correctly when using the Smith Machine**—this makes all the difference in the world regarding the amount of effectiveness and type of adaptation you are targeting. For standard squats, you want your feet slightly forward of the bar—not right under it. Your knees will let you know what feels correct here. You can also use some foot positions that would be difficult with free weight squats, such as feet together or as wide as the machine uprights allow. Try them all.

- Two intensity techniques work particularly well with any form of Smith Machine squat—heavy partials and strip sets—and you don't need a spotter to use them. No excuses here.

- Besides standard squats, you can also effectively perform front and bench squats on the Smith Machine.

Bench Squats

- If you've never done them, bench squats can be effective for increasing power at the bottom of the squat, teaching the bottom pause, teaching proper depth, and performing partial reps. The key here is selection of appropriate bench heights.

- Most gyms only have stand-alone flat benches that you can use for bench squats. Unfortunately, most of these benches place you just above parallel when your butt touches the bench. This is good for performing heavy partials or boosting your ego, but not so good for just about everything else mentioned above. Hopefully, your gym has a set of plyometric benches of varying heights you can choose from. You want three benches—one that places you just below parallel, one at parallel and another just above parallel. If you work diligently on all three, your regular free weight squats will accelerate in performance.

- **A warning about bench squats**—don't come landing down on the bench forcefully—you want a very light touch and go movement. Any sudden landing on the bench can cause severe spinal compression from both ends—remember, you've got resistance at both ends here, so be careful. You don't want to give yourself a stinger, or worse.

Trap Bar Squats

- If you have access to a Trap Bar, this is an excellent way to occasionally shock your quads by taking them to complete (and I mean complete) failure, while sparing your lower back. Since the weight is not supported by your back and is at the center point of your body (on each side), you can literally keep squatting until you can't get another rep, without fear of falling over. If you have a partner, he or she can also strip some weight off after you fail so that you can continue your misery and take those quads to new levels of pumpitude. This is the same technique as used with belt squats.

● Use this exercise if you are recovering from low back issues. Don't use this exercise as a weekly staple—that's what the squats are for.

Leg Presses

● Leg press machines come in three flavors, all based on the angle of attack: vertical, 45°, and horizontal. The closer the leg press is to vertical, the more effective it is. Since the vertical leg press seems to be relegated to the dust bin of history, your gym is more likely to have either the 45° or horizontal leg press, or both. Opt for the 45° version, unless you are recovering from a lower back injury.

● Foot placement is paramount here. You don't want your feet too high (danger of rounding the lower back), nor too low (too much knee stress). Either position your feet pointing straight ahead or angle them out slightly, depending on whether your foot stance is narrow, normal or wide.

● Try alternating between normal, wide, and narrow foot stances from set to set or workout to workout for optimal results on this machine.

● **Every so often, perform leg presses one leg at a time.** This more intense version of leg presses will help you identify and correct imbalances in strength.

● If you are having low back issues, use the horizontal leg press, since this version of the press puts the least amount of stress on the lower back, especially if you can adjust the seat so that the range of motion is decreased somewhat.

Lunges and Adductor Machines

- I'm not a big fan of lunges or the adductor machines. You can build just as muscular and shapely legs with various squats, leg presses, and extensions.

- **Both barbell and dumbbell lunges are useful for enhancing stability and balance.** The dumbbell version is easier to perform and will allow you to lunge across the gym without taking out everyone in your way, including yourself. They can also be useful for placing additional stress on the glutes, depending upon stride length and depth.

- The Adductor Machine is typically used by women, although with heavy weight, men can use it effectively to build inner quads. However, you can obtain superior results by performing all varieties of wide-stance squats instead.

- **The most effective use of the Adductor Machine is to help correct the inward knee motion that many have when squatting.** This motion is indicative of weak inner thighs and heavy weight on the Adductor Machine can help correct that over time.

Hamstrings

Curls the leg back.

Key Exercises	Stiff Leg Deadlifts w/Barbell, Lying Leg Curls
Alternate Exercises	Seated Leg Curls, Standing Leg Curls, Reverse Lunges

General Tips

- **Separate your hamstring workout from your quad workout, if possible**. Otherwise, your hamstring workout may suffer, due to fatigue, especially of the lower back. Since stiff-leg deadlifts are one of the best hamstring mass builders, you need your lower back to be strong.

- **You build big hamstrings with stiff-leg deadlifts, not leg curls.** Read that last sentence again.

- **It's a good idea to alternate starting your hamstring workouts between leg curls and stiff-leg deadlifts.** This tends to keep the hamstrings adapting and growing. Give yourself a break from stiff-leg deadlifts once every four workouts and just concentrate on leg curls that day. Over the years, your lower back will reward you for this.

- **Every so often, you may find it useful to superset leg curls immediately after every set for quads.** This will accomplish three things: 1) you'll end up doing a lot more sets for hamstrings than you normally do, thus providing a volume effect; 2) you'll be able to keep the weight much higher for more sets on leg curls than you normally do, and; 3) your hamstrings will be sore as hell for the next few days. Have fun sitting.

- **For most people, hamstring development lags behind the development of the quads**—relatively speaking. By relative, what you want to see is approximately a 60%/40% split between your total leg mass of quads-to-hamstrings. When you start getting muscular imbalances of 70% quads to 30% hamstrings, that's when you start to run into problems such as pulled hamstrings, hamstring tears, etc. Remember the general rule for legs: if your upper leg mass is 60/40 quads/hamstrings and you really develop your calves, then your overall leg appearance should be very good. Keep this in mind ladies.

- **If your hamstrings are lagging, three good strategies for improving them are**: 1) superset them with every set of quads, as described above; 2) work them separately before quads, in addition to working them on another day, and; 3) if working them on their own day, add a few more sets (10-12).

Stiff-Leg Deadlifts

- **Stiff-leg deadlifts are the king of hamstring builders.** Most people don't do them or do them wrong, but do them you must if you want exceptional legs. I can walk into any gym and pick out the guys (and gals) who do this exercise regularly and those that don't.

- The best visualization I know for this exercise is to imagine that a fisherman has cast his line right into your buttocks and is reeling you in from 50 feet away. Your rear end should be traveling straight backward which causes your hamstrings to stretch. Continue until your hamstrings are completely stretched, with your back remaining flat (not rounded). Then, return to the starting position in exactly the same manner—rear end pushing straight forward until you are upright. If you do this correctly, your hamstrings should be sore the next day, but your lower back should not. That's when you know you have this exercise down. Don't worry, it may take awhile, but with continual practice and concentration you will get it.

- **You can perform these with a barbell, dumbbells, cables, a Smith Machine or a Trap Bar**, although by now, you should know that the barbell is the preferred method for building mass quickly.

- The advantage to using dumbbells, two cables or the Trap Bar is that the weight can be kept to your sides, thus reducing the stress on the lower back. The dumbbells and cables will also allow you to perform drop-sets easily, which will make things hard ☺.

● **Using a Smith Machine can also help those with lower back issues**, since stability becomes less of an issue. The Smith Machine also lets you perform drop-sets effectively—something not as easily done with a barbell. Try placing two 10lb plates on the floor where your toes would rest while performing this exercise. Then, place your toes on the plates and do the exercise. You should notice that your hamstrings get a little bit of a pre-stretch where they attach behind the knees with this technique.

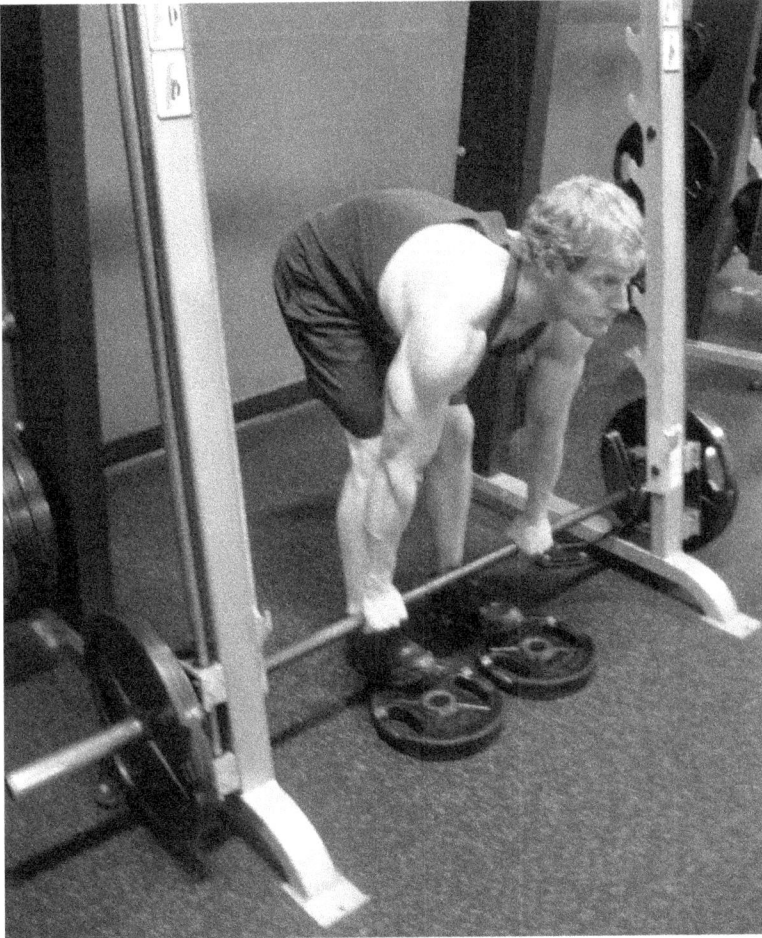

Smith Machine Stiff-Leg Deadlifts—note the toes on the plates

● Remember, you should use the three foot width variations (narrow, normal, wide) on this exercise and note the results. Perform this exercise on the floor, not on a bench as some bodybuilding magazines and books illustrate.

- **Keep your feet pointed straight ahead when doing these—not outward.** You can also try pointing your feet ever so slightly inward—and I mean almost imperceptibly inward. I find this helps to keep everything locked into place during the movement.

Leg Curls

- Leg curls are the lower body equivalent of preacher (lying and seated leg curls) or spider curls (standing leg curls) for your biceps. This makes sense, especially since these two body parts share similar anatomical and motor precepts. They don't call hamstrings the *biceps femoris* for nothing.

- You can perform leg curls lying, seated or standing. No matter which type you choose, leg curls present a good opportunity to employ several intensity techniques, especially 21s, drop sets, burns, partials, and wave sets. Additionally, you can perform these curls one leg at a time, and discover if one hamstring is weaker than the other is—then correct that imbalance.

- Make sure you vary the width of your thighs when performing lying or seated leg curls. Try a few sets with your thighs together when you curl, and a few as far apart as the bench/seat will allow. Note the difference in feel. Incorporate both width variations into your workout regimen.

- One variation of lying leg curls that is particularly painful, yet effective, is what I call Concentration Lying Leg Curls. Here's how to do it. Lie down on the bench as normal. Then, using your arms to support your upper body, lift your upper body up until it forms a straight line with your lower body on the machine. Keeping that position throughout, curl the weight. You'll find that this form of the exercise precludes you from using anywhere near the amount of weight you can normally do. You'll also notice that nothing but hamstring is involved—and the lactic acid building up real fast. Have fun—this will really make your hamstrings pop out.

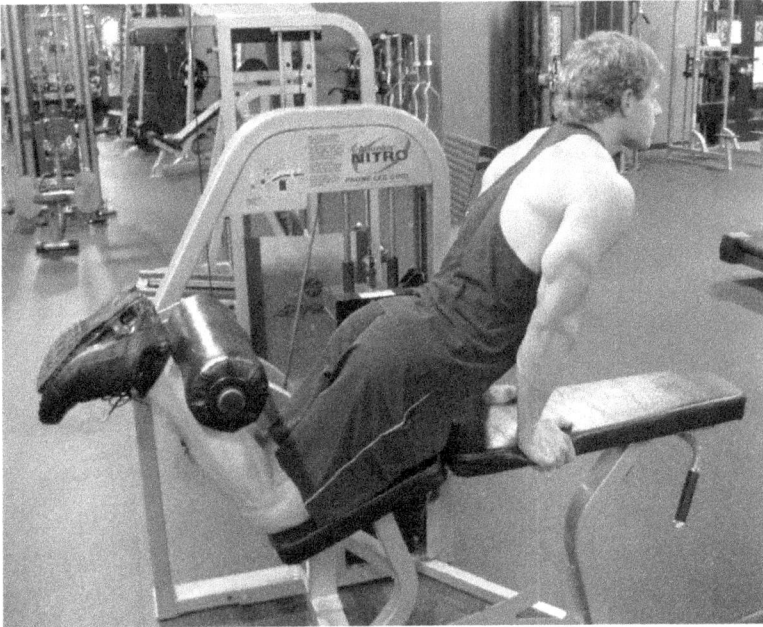

Concentration Leg Curls

Hamstrings

Calves

Flexes the foot.

Key Exercises	Standing Calf Raises, Seated Calf Raises, Donkey Calf Raises, Calf Presses
Alternate Exercises	Jumping Squats

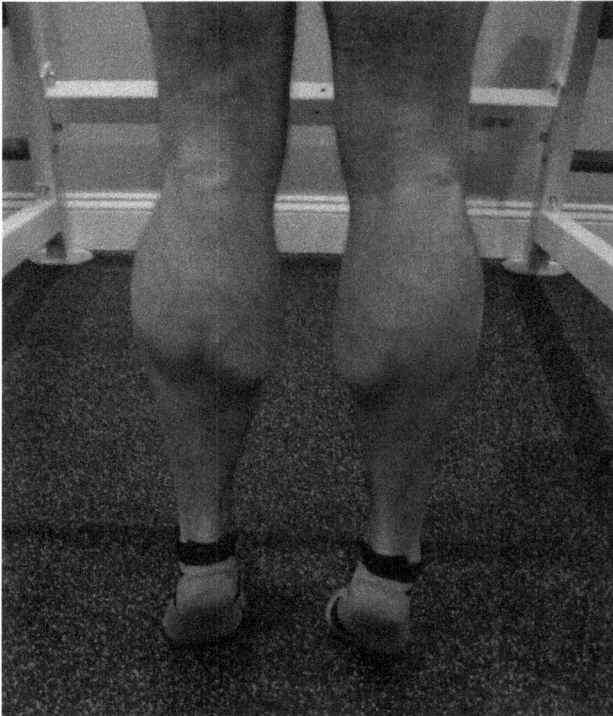

General Tips

● Although genetics play a large role in your overall calf size potential, consistent use of the tips in this section, coupled with the various intensity techniques presented later will produce good results. There is a direct relation between calf results and the workload/effort you put into them. Treat them as first-class citizens and they will respond. Do them often, do them heavy, do them high rep and low rep, and do them first.

- **Range of motion is essential with calf work—maybe more so than with any other body part.** That's because when you walk around every day you are working your calves, but only through a partial range of motion. Make your calves work through the other two extremes in the full range (full stretch and full extension) and that's where they really start to grow—you'll feel it the next day. Believe me. Calf soreness is one of the most excruciatingly good pain sensations you'll get out of the gym. Hurts so good.

- Because range of motion is so critical with calf work, donkey calf raises work better than any type of standing raise due to the pre-stretch that occurs when performing this exercise.

- Ask any gym member and most trainers—why are there both seated and standing calf raise machines? Most people don't know. Your calf complex consists primarily of two muscles: the gastrocnemius (gastroc) and the soleus. Since the gastroc attaches behind your knee at the top, you need to keep your leg straight to work this muscle through its full range of motion—thus, the standing machine. The soleus attaches below the knee, which means you don't need to be standing at all to work this one through the full range—thus, the seated machine—because as we all know, given a choice between standing and sitting, modern man likes to sit. Make sure your calf workouts include both types of raises if you want complete calf development—those with legs straight and bent.

- **In addition to full range of motion, foot stance width is important to complete calf development as well.** Your gastrocs are comprised of two vertical muscles, one on the outer half and one on the inner half. Many weight lifting aficionados will direct you to perform your calf work with your toes turned inward or outward in order to hit the inner or outer gastroc head. Your calves don't work this way. You just need to rise all the way up on your toes and descend into a full stretch. However, how far apart you have your feet does make a big difference. Here's why. Try this experiment. Stand in bare feet, put your feet a little wider than shoulder width apart and rise up on your toes. Notice how your foot tends to shift your weight onto your big toes? Feel that inner gastroc head contract? Now, put your feet together and try the same thing. Your weight shifts to your pinkie toes, doesn't it? Feel that outer calf head contract? That's how you should perform calf raises, whether standing or sitting. Do some of your raise with your feet close together and others farther apart. Change from set to set or from workout to workout. It's up to you. Just don't use the same stance all the time. This should be sounding familiar by now.

● Your calves will get indirect work when performing squats and deadlifts. The heavier you go in those exercises, the bigger your calves will get.

Standing Calf Raises

● Besides the typical standing calf raise machine found in most gyms, there are several other ways to perform this type of exercise: standing on one-leg with a dumbbell, with a hack squat machine, standing with a barbell, using a Smith Machine, etc.

● Many standing calf raise machines in gyms are poorly designed. You should be completely perpendicular to the floor at all times when standing on the foot platform. Typically, the engineering on these machines has you leaning forward while performing the exercise, since the shoulder pads do not extend to the same plane as the foot platform. In these cases, you may find it better to turn around and do the exercise backwards on the machine, with your back facing the weight stack. Try it and see how it feels.

● **One-leg calf raises holding a dumbbell are a good exercise for determining imbalances in calf weakness, as well as correcting those weaknesses.** Any time you perform unilateral exercises, the intensity automatically ratchets up. Use the spotting platform at the back of bench press or shoulder press stations for this exercise. If one of your calves is smaller/weaker than the other, do some extra sets of this exercise with only that calf, before your regular calf workout.

● **If you want to work old school and improve your athleticism, try standing calf raises with a barbell.** Use the squat rack, step out as if you are going to do a squat and start doing calf raises. You'll find balance to be your first challenge, but over time you'll really learn to feel everything that's going on below your knees. For additional challenge, place two 25lb plates on the floor and stand with your toes on them so that you get a stretch and bigger range of motion—but be careful— you're a weight lifter, not a Cirque du Soleil performer. For those not wishing to perform this high-wire act, you can use the Smith Machine instead.

● **You can also perform standing calf raises on the Hack Squat machine.** Based on the design of the machine at your gym, you can either stand as you would at the top of a hack squat and rise up on your toes, or turn around and face the pad on the machine and do it that way. In addition, placing 25lb plates on the foot platform will allow you to get a little stretch at the bottom. This type of calf raise really teaches you to get as high as possible on your toes.

Donkey Calf Raises

● **Although this exercise may be embarrassing for some, continued use of it will produce results that will embarrass others.** It is probably the most effective exercise for the gastrocs due to the extreme range of motion you get here.

● **If your gym has a Donkey Calf Raise machine, consider yourself blessed.** Otherwise, you'll have to improvise. Here's how. You need a willing participant (the heavier, the better) and a Smith Machine. Set the bar of the machine just below waist level. Grab a pair of 25lb plates (an aerobic floor bench is even better) and place them a few inches apart on the floor, a couple feet back from the bar (you'll need to fine tune the placement of the plates for your body). Placing your forearms on the bar, bend over at the waist until your upper body is parallel to the floor. Now, ask your participant to climb onto your hips, like they are preparing to ride you in the Belmont. They can use the support bars of the Smith Machine for balance. Then, standing with your toes on the plates you placed on the floor, rise up as high as you can, squeeze and lower slowly into the stretch. If you need additional resistance, have your partner hold a heavy dumbbell or plate.

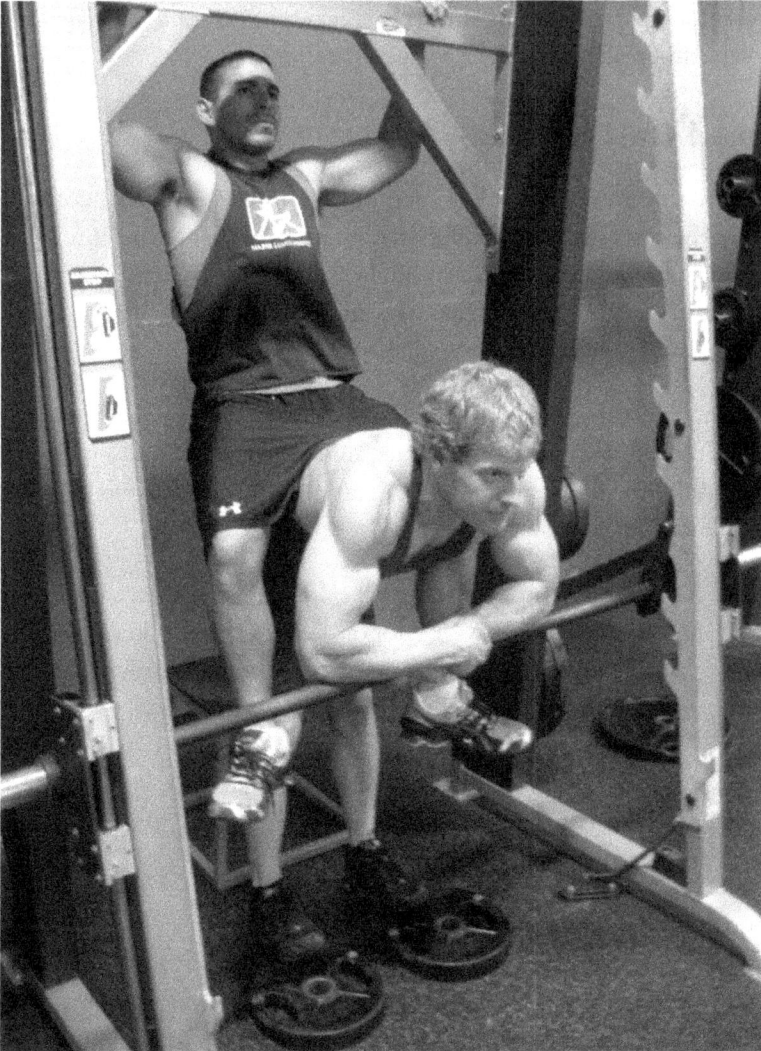

Smith Machine Donkey Calf Raises—might look stupid, but are highly effective

Calf Presses

● **Calf presses on a leg press machine are a good, albeit inferior second cousin to standing calf raises**, since gravity does not have a direct line on you. Here, you can use a god-awful amount of weight, but that's where most make their mistake. Use calf presses to really accentuate the amount of stretch you get at the bottom. Over time, keep this form up and the weight will go up and up.

Seated Calf Raises

- **Seated calf raises provide a gladiatorial arena for mental combat—** since the soleus really responds well to very high rep ranges through a full range of motion, you'll need to hunker down and see how far you can push it past the lactic acid pain barrier. If you make it to the other side, large, diamond-shaped calves will be yours.

- When you work the soleus muscles of your calf (remember: bent-knee), you have a few options besides the standard seated calf raise machine. You can perform them one-leg at a time, seated with a barbell or dumbbells, or even squatted down.

- Ever wonder what those guys from the 50s did before seated calf raise machines were invented? Well, a lot of them just didn't do calves, but those that did, sat their ass down on a bench with a barbell or dumbbells resting on their knees and did toes raises. It's still effective today. Try placing an aerobic bench or 25lb plates on the floor to rest your toes on. Make sure your lower leg is completely perpendicular to the floor throughout the entire range of motion. You may also need a folded towel over your knees for protection.

- Squatting calf raises. Never heard of them you say? Try this. After each set of seated calf raises on the machine, grab onto a sturdy upright, put your feet together and squat down until your hamstrings touch your calves. Now, using only your calves, rise up on your toes, hold the contraction for a second, and then go back down. Do about 25-50 of these and tell me if your calves aren't literally on fire. This will give you incredible calf delineation from the side

Intensity Techniques

Eventually, even the best of us will reach a (temporary?) limit to how much weight we are able to lift in a particular exercise. You need to change something to make the muscle grow. That's where intensity techniques come into play.

There are a myriad of intensity enhancing techniques you can apply to your workouts. This section talks about the most effective ones (in alphabetical order).

21's

This technique consists of a set of 21 reps, performed in three segments—the first seven reps through the beginning half of the movement, the second seven through the second half of the movement, and the final seven through the full range.

Most likely, you've done these with curls for your biceps, but they are equally as effective on most other exercises, especially lying leg curls (hey, they are pretty much like your biceps), side lateral raises, calf raises, and squats.

Hey, who says you have to limit yourself to 21 reps? You can use the same technique for 12s, 15s, or 18s. Start with the second half of the movement as the first seven reps. Go crazy.

5 Sets of 5

This is a good technique to build strength with basic, compound exercises like bench presses, deadlifts, and squats. But don't necessarily limit yourself to those—try this on bent-over rows, barbell curls, and leg curls.

10 sets of 10

If 5 Sets of 5 are good, then 10 Sets of 10 must be better—right? Maybe. Depends on what you are looking for. Unlike 5 Sets of 5, this technique is optimized to build muscular size, not just pure strength, and you can use this on any type of exercise effectively.

You haven't really squatted until you've done 10 sets of 10. That's like a rite of passage or trial by fire for true iron warriors. They don't call this technique

German Volume Training for nothing. So, go make yourself some legs like a female East German athlete of yesteryear.

Addition Sets

Addition Sets are the opposite of Drop Sets. With this technique, you start with a relatively light weight for high reps (12-15) to failure, and subsequently add weight with lower reps (6-10) to failure on progressive sets. Unlike the traditional Pyramid technique, you perform each set to failure, even with the lighter weights. Therefore, it's essential that you choose your weights wisely.

Addition Sets work particularly well for denser fiber groups, such as calves and forearms, which tend to recover quickly between sets.

Alternating Sets

With this technique, you alternate between two antagonistic exercises, using the same rest periods as Straight Sets. Alternating Sets allow you to use more weight (and generate a greater workload) by regulating fatigue across body parts.

Some good examples of Alternating Sets are:

- Inclines Presses / Chins
- Curls / Pushdowns
- Chins / Dips
- Squats / Leg Curls

Remember, after the first exercise in the Alternating Set, you take your normal rest period, then do the second exercise, then rest, and repeat the process.

Alternating Sets are similar to Antagonistic Supersets, except for the rest period between exercises.

Ascending Sets

You're familiar with these. Think back to when you just started lifting weights. Pick a target number of reps, such as eight, and continue to perform that number of reps for every set, while progressively increasing the weight each set.

Ascending Sets are the most popular method of performing set progression and is the standard method of resistance training. It also forms the basis of strength training used in Olympic lifting and power lifting.

If you haven't done these in awhile, it's probably time to revisit them.

Burns

Burns are small, short-range movements, typically performed at the end of a set, when the muscle(s) have exhausted from full range of motion movement. They are typically performed in the stretch or contracted positions of the movement. This technique helps you to recruit additional muscle fibers once you can't perform a full rep anymore.

Some good exercises for burns include preacher curls, calf raises (any type), leg curls, and leg extensions. They really work well for biceps, calves, and hamstrings.

You'll note that most of these are not compound-multi joint movements—there's a reason for this—burns can be dangerous in those movements. That doesn't mean you can't try them, but I would recommend doing them on a Smith Machine or in a power rack. However, be careful with burns in the stretch position, especially with preacher curls—you don't want to hyperextend your elbow or strain your lower biceps attachment. Always remain in control of the lowering of a weight.

Cheating

The key to cheating is knowing how and when to cheat. And by cheating, we're talking about deviating from strict exercise form here, nothing else.

A cheat rep is a rep that deviates from strict form, such as leaning, using momentum, etc., which allows you to continue the set after you can't do another rep with strict form.

There are two keys to using this technique correctly. The first is to use just the minimal amount of deviation from strict form as necessary in order to complete the rep. You should always be striving to eliminate the cheat from the rep when you are using this technique. And the second is to only use cheat reps AFTER you can't complete another rep in strict form (there is an exception to this—see below). Don't be a lemming like most guys in the gym where their entire workout seems to consist of cheat reps. You can tell who does this just by looking at them. Their physique is a big sloppy mess, just like their form.

Occasionally, cheating can be used for an entire set or series of sets, in order to attempt to break through plateaus. Cheat Curls are a perfect example of this. Just don't keep using this technique workout after workout or you'll start morphing into that big sloppy mess I mentioned.

Besides curls, cheating works well with pushdowns, push presses, standing calf raises and lat pulldowns.

Compound Sets

This one is simple: two or more exercises for the same body part with minimal rest between sets. Pick two exercises with this technique and you have a superset. Pick three, and you've got a tri-set. Pick more than three and it's called a giant set.

Here's some examples:

Abs (Giant Set): Reverse Crunches, Crunches, Twists, Side Bends

Biceps (Superset): Barbell Curls, Dumbbell Hammer Curls

Down the Rack

This technique is the same as Drop Sets, except it's performed with dumbbells or fixed barbells. Pick your starting weight, go to failure, pick up a lighter weight, go to failure, etc. Little to no rest between weight drops as you go down the dumbbell/barbell rack. Also known as "running the rack". Use this when you want to flush a lot of blood into a specific area.

This one is good for curls, laterals, overhead extensions, presses, flys, and shrugs.

Drop Sets

Drop sets require you to perform a set of an exercise to failure (or just short of failure), then reduce the weight somewhat and continue the set for more reps. This technique is designed to build muscle mass, and is not as effective for building strength, power, or speed.

The theory behind Drop Sets is that even though you may have reached a point of positive muscular failure, you may not have activated all your muscle fiber types in that area. You can recruit additional muscle fibers by continuing the set through by reducing the weight, thus increasing the stress and overload placed on the muscle, forcing adaptation to occur. It's all about adaptation, baby.

So, one big question you may have is—how much should I drop the weight each time? Good question. A good starting average is to reduce the weight about 15% for each "drop", although the real answer is you'll need to experiment to find out the best amount based on your current capabilities. Over time, you may find that your drop weight percentage goes down, since your muscular endurance is getting better.

In order to maximize the efficiency of drop sets, keep these key points in mind:

- **Set Up Your Equipment in Advance**

- **Keep Rest Intervals to a Minimum** (0-10 seconds)

  Remember, the shorter the rest interval, the higher the intensity.

- **Perform Two Weight Drops** (most of the time)

- **Perform 6-12 Reps Per Drop** (most of the time)

- **Use Drop Sets Sparingly**

  The 3:1 Method is a good rule of thumb here—either perform one drop set for every three straight sets, or use drop-setting once every four workouts.

Finally, there are many variations of Drop Sets, which I'll discuss below:

Ascending Drop Sets

Decrease the weight by a substantial amount and increase the number of reps at each drop. A typical rep pattern here is 6-12-20 (6 reps with initial weight, 12 reps after first drop, 20 reps with final drop).

Descending Drop Sets (Tight Drop Sets)

Decrease the weight by a small amount so that the number of reps at each drop decreases. A typical rep pattern here is 12-8-4-2. This is an example of a Tight Drop Set.

Down the Rack

We discussed this one above. Here, it's just Drop Sets with dumbbells or fixed barbells—no unloading of plates.

Drop Supersets

This variation uses two exercises, where you alternate between the exercises while reducing the weight on both—get ready for a marathon.

Some ideas here include:

Chest: Dumbbell Flys + Barbell Presses

Shoulders: Dumbbell Laterals + Dumbbell Presses

Biceps: Barbell Curls + Dumbbell Concentration Curls

Those are just a few examples. Really, just pick any two exercises for the same body part and alternate between them. That's it. Anything goes.

Grip/Stance Change Drop Sets

Change your grip or foot stance width between each weight drop. The purpose here is to subject the muscle(s) to stress from differing angles and load patterns.

This one is really effective with barbell rows, bench presses, curls, squats, leg presses and leg extensions.

Halves

Reduce the weight by 50% between drops. This will let you start with a heavy weight that you can only get for a few reps, and lets you keep going into the higher reps as the weight lightens.

Halves work really well for the big lifts, like squats, presses and rows. Also, try them with curls, pushdowns, lateral raises and calf raises (your calves will love you for this one).

Machine Drop Sets

Pretty easy to figure this one out, right? Drop sets using a machine with a weight stack. Just pull the pin for each drop. Doesn't get much easier than that—which is why they are a perfect introduction to the world of intensity training for beginners.

Power Drop Sets

This variation combines heavy weights, low reps, and small drops in weight (10-15%). Try to keep the reps at six on each drop and just do two drops.

If you did this twice for bench presses, it would look like this:

Barbell Bench Press: (275x6 > 245x6 > 205x6) x 2

Wait a minute—what's that notation above? That's LiftScript™. I'll get to that in a moment.

Rest-Pause Drop Sets

Rest for a fixed number of seconds (five, ten, or fifteen) between drops. This allows your muscles to slightly recover—therefore, you can use more weight with this technique, which is why it's good for increasing strength and size.

Strip Sets

Drop sets with barbells, where the plates are "stripped" off as the set progresses.

Try this one with presses, starting with a bunch of 10lb plates on each side of the bar. Man, that bar is going to be heavy when all the plates are removed.

Wide Drop Sets

This variation refers to large weight reductions between drops. Wide drop sets are typically easier to perform than Tight Drop Sets, since they allow you to perform higher reps. Due to the higher reps and subsequent cardiovascular fatigue, Wide Drop Sets are particularly useful for exercises that work large muscle groups, such as chest, back and legs.

Try these with bench presses, squats, and leg presses.

Here's an example of a Wide Drop Set:

Barbell Bench Press: 275x5 > 225x12 > 135x20

Fixed Time Sets

Perform an exercise for a fixed number of minutes, taking very brief rest intervals (15-30 seconds) between sets of muscular failure. When the time period is over, then the exercise is complete.

Here's an example with Seated Calf Raises:

You decide to use a Fixed Time Set of 5 minutes with break intervals of 30 seconds when failure occurs. Start the set, noting the start time. Continue until you can't do another rep and rack the weight. Wait 30 seconds. Now do your next set until failure. Wait 30 seconds. Continue like this until 5 minutes are up. Congratulations—you just performed the 5 Minute Calves routine (more on this later), which uses Fixed Time Sets. Now, try getting up and walking...

Besides calves, Fixed Time Sets work really well with curls and pushdowns. See what else works for you.

Forced Reps

You need a good spotter for this one—and the key here is a **good** spotter (why are they so hard to find?). With Forced Reps, the spotter should provide only *minimal* assistance when you are nearing positive muscular failure—just enough to keep the weight moving through the range of motion. On some unilateral exercises, such as Dumbbell Preacher Curls, a spotter is not necessarily required, as you can use your other hand to assist with the forced reps.

Properly performed forced reps are very demanding on the body and can severely tax your recovery system. Therefore, only use them periodically, both within workouts and between workouts. Don't be one of those guys who not only performs a 1RM on bench presses every workout, but wants some forced reps as well.

Given that warning, Forced Reps are a very effective method for breaking through training plateaus and promoting progress. You can use this technique with almost any exercise effectively; however, you might want to think twice about doing them with squats or deadlifts. You have been warned—again.

Giant Sets

Four or more exercises performed one after the other, without rest between exercises.

Typically, all the exercises in a Giant Set target the same body part—however, this technique works well for antagonistic body parts (biceps/triceps, chest/back, quads/hamstrings). Also, there is no reason you can't perform the same exercise more than once within a Giant Set. You make the rules.

Here's a sample Giant Set for back:

Chins + Bent-over Barbell Rows + Pulldown + Seated Cable Rows + Stiff-Arm Lat Pushdowns

Variations of Giant Sets

There are two specific variations of Giant Sets you might find useful:

Perform Exercises in Order of Range of Motion Stress

Here, you perform the exercises in the order of the stress area placed on the muscle group, from the stretch position, to midrange, to the contracted position.

For example, a Giant Set performed this way for biceps would look something like this:

Barbell Preacher Curls (stretch) + Barbell Curls (midrange) + Cable Concentration Curls (contraction)

Single Exercise/Multiple Variations

Here, you perform a single exercise, but use multiple variations from the mechanically weakest to the strongest.

For example, a Giant Set performed this way for back would look something like this:

Wide-Grip Pulldowns (weakest mechanical position)   +
Wide-Grip Neutral Pulldowns   +
Parallel-Grip Pulldowns   +
Reverse-Grip Pulldowns (strongest mechanical position)

Halves (50% Drop Sets)

The "halving method" is a variation of Drop Sets, except you only reduce the weight one time and you reduce it by 50%.

Halves allow you to use two differing rep ranges and muscle fiber types within a single set. Typically, the starting weight should be something that you will fail on around the 6th rep, and after cutting the weight in half, you should be able to get about 20 reps—however, these are just guidelines—don't stop just because you got the 6 or the 20 reps. Choose your weights wisely.

This technique is very easy to perform with weight machines, since you only need to move the pin up the stack to decrease the weight in half.

Negatives

This technique concentrates on the eccentric (lowering) phase of the exercise. It's typical to perform Negatives at the end of a set, when your muscles have failed from performing the exercise. However, you can perform Negatives effectively as standalone sets.

There are a couple points to keep in mind in order to perform Negatives effectively:

- Use a weight that's about 10% heavier than your 1RM on the exercise

- Use a good spotter, unless you have a death wish.

- Actively resist the lowering of the weight the entire time.

- The negative rep should take about 5-10 seconds to lower—if it goes down faster than that on the first negative then the weight is too heavy.

- Try to perform negatives near the beginning of your workouts (after warm-ups and some working sets, of course) when you are at full energy.

- Don't perform negatives at every workout, since they can create extreme stress on the body (use the 3:1 Method here). This technique will test your body's recovery ability to the limit.

- Don't perform negatives unless you are an advanced weightlifter.

Another method of performing negatives is to have your spotter add plates or provide manual resistance on the eccentric portion of the movement—but you really better trust your spotter for this or injury may result.

Finally, you can perform negatives effectively on weight-stack machines since you can quickly adjust the weight via the selector pin and use just one limb (leg or arm) to lower the weight.

Partials

Partial reps (Partials) use only a limited range of the full range of motion for an exercise. This should allow you to use more weight than normal, thus increasing the stress on the muscle as well as helping to build stronger connective tissue (tendons and ligaments). Along with Negatives, they are very effective for breaking through sticking points.

Partials can be performed anywhere within an exercise's range of motion— get creative with this. You can also perform them at the end of a set, when you can't do another full range of motion with the exercise.

So, what's a good number of partials to perform at the end of a set? Try for 3-6 and see how that works for you.

Some good examples of using partials include:

- **Biceps**: At the end of your set of curls by performing just the bottom part of the curl.

- **Triceps**: At the end of your set of pushdowns by performing just the first half of the motion.

- **Back**: I don't recommend the use of partial movements for the back, other than partial deadlifts in a rack. The back really needs full range of motion to grow to its full potential.

- **Chest**: Set the pins in the power rack or Smith Machine so that you are only performing the top part of the press—or the mid-range of the press—or the start of the press. You get the idea. By the way, this is a good way to increase your bench press.

- **Delts**: At the end of your set of side laterals by raising the dumbbells as high as you can and holding each partial rep.

- **Quads**: Set the pins in the power rack or Smith Machine so that you are only performing the top part of the squat.

- **Hamstrings**: At the end of your set of leg curls by performing just the first half of the motion.

- **Calves**: At the end of your set of calf raises/presses by performing just the bottom half of the motion. For seated raises, try performing just the top half of the motion.

Pre-Exhaustion

A superset for a single muscle group, with the first exercise an isolation (single-joint) movement and the second a compound (multi-joint) movement.

The goal here is to fatigue the target muscle group with the isolation exercise, then switch to the compound exercise, which employs assistance muscles to exhaust the area completely.

You typically see this performed with chest (fly/press) and quads (extension/squat), although you can use it with any muscle group. For example, a typical pre-exhaust set for chest would have you do dumbbell flys followed up with dumbbell presses. As your chest gets tired from the flys, you switch to presses, which now uses your triceps to help you complete each rep. Notice that this is completely opposite of what typically happens when you perform presses for your chest—your triceps tend to tire out before your chest does, right? Pre-Exhaustion throws this in reverse.

The big disadvantage to Pre-Exhaustion training is that you won't be able to use your normal heavier weights on the second exercise, since your target muscle is already fatigued from the isolation movement. Therefore, don't use this technique as the basis for your workouts. It's meant to be used sparingly, like most of the other techniques in this section.

The table below gives you some good Pre-Exhaust exercise combos:

Muscle Group	Pre-Exhaust Exercise Combos
Biceps	Concentrations Curls > Barbell Curls
Back	Pullovers > Chins or Pulldown
	Pullovers > Rows
Chest	Flys > Presses
	Flys > Dips
Delts	Laterals > Presses
Quads	Leg Extensions > Squats or Leg Presses
Traps	Shrugs > Upright Rows
Triceps	Pushdowns > Dips
	French Press > Close-Grip Bench Press

Pyramids

Increase the weight and decrease the reps on each subsequent set for a body part. Besides Straight Sets, this is probably the most common weightlifting technique performed—you'll see it in every weight lifting book and gym in the world. However, don't forget there are a couple useful versions of Pyramids:

Half Pyramids

This is the most commonly performed type of Pyramid—increase the weight and decrease the reps on each set for a body part. Really helps you acclimate to the movement and warm-up your muscles and your psyche in preparation for the really big weights and lower reps as you climb the pyramid.

Here's a typical Half Pyramid for Bench Presses:

135x15, 185x12, 225x10, 245x8, 275x6, 295x4

You've done that before, right? Thought so.

Full Pyramids

By now, you can probably guess what this one entails. You go up the pyramid, then reverse yourself and come back down the same way you went up.

Here's a typical Full Pyramid for Bench Presses:

135x15, 185x12, 225x10, 245x8, 275x6, 295x4, 275x6, 245x8, 225x10, 185x12, 135x15

Not quite as commonly performed as Half Pyramids, but useful if you need to add more volume into your workout and don't want to waste your time with cable crossovers or talking about mortgage rates.

Inverted Pyramids

This is the most intense type of Pyramid training. After a few warm-up sets, go right to your heaviest weight. On the following sets, reduce the weight, but keep increasing the number of reps. Then, you can opt to go back up the inverted pyramid by increasing the weight/decreasing the reps on the following sets. Choose your weights wisely here.

Here's an Inverted Pyramid for Bench Presses (after the warm-up sets):

295x4, 275x6, 245x8, 225x10, 185x12, 225x10, 245x8, 275x6, 295x4

Rep Targeting

With this technique, the goal is to reach a certain "target" number of total reps, no matter how many sets it takes to get there. This works best when you are using your body weight or a constant exercise weight. Of course, your goal over time should be to reduce the number of sets it takes you to reach your target number of reps. This one will test your fortitude.

For example, let's say you target 50 reps for Chins using your body weight. On your first set, you get 17 reps. Now, you have 33 reps remaining. On the next set, you get 13. That leaves you with 20 reps to go. Eventually, you reach the 50 reps after five sets. Pretty good. Now, try to do it next time in four sets—or with some weight hanging from you. Good luck.

Here's another example using Squats. Your target is 100 reps. You set the barbell to 225lbs. On your first set you churn out 21 reps. Nice—just 79 to go. Eventually, after you think you are going to die several times over, you get to that elusive 100 reps in nine sets. Just making it through that gauntlet is a mental accomplishment few others even attempt. Congratulations—your legs just got bigger. Now do it again next time in eight sets.

Rest-Pause

This technique allows you to extend a set by taking very short rest breaks (5-15 seconds) between reps as you approach failure. In practice, performing two rest-pauses during your set should work best.

Although you'll typically use this technique as you approach failure, you can also use it right from the onset of a set, in order to handle some really heavy weights.

Here's an example of a Rest-Pause set of bench presses: 225x8+2+1

In this example, we did 8 reps with 225, racked the bar for about 10 seconds, did another 2 reps, racked it again, and then did a final rep, for a total of 11 reps in the rest-pause set. Much more intense than if we just did 225 for 8 reps and ended the set.

Same Weight Progression

Use the same weight for a specific number of reps on each set of an exercise.

You can expand this technique in order to obtain intensity benefits as an advanced lifter by using these variations:

Same Reps

Here you not only use the same weight on each set, but you also try to get the same number of reps on each. Sound familiar? It's part of the core of progressive resistance training—and it gets hard real fast, especially as you increase the volume of sets.

Ascending Reps

Here, you consistently use the same weight, but more reps on each set. Sounds easy, but just try it. Depending on how wisely you've chosen your weight, you'll either feel like a fool or a genius at the end.

Descending Reps

This variation has you using the same weight, with fewer reps on each set. Huh? Sounds easy. Yeah, but try it with a weight that you can do about 12-15 reps with on the first set and go from there. This technique is very useful if you have a tendon, muscle or joint that you are in the process of healing from an injury.

Static Holds

This technique is as much for your mind as your body and is one of the places where you confront your fear. It's simple. After a couple of regular sets of an exercise, pick a weight heavier than anything you've ever done on that exercise. Then, just hold it in the contracted position as long as possible.

Static Holds will help to build connective tissue strength, increase muscle density and improve your confidence with heavy weights. You can also use this technique at various stages of an exercise's range of motion in order to break through performance plateaus.

Best used with compound, multi-joint movements such as presses, squats, deadlifts and dips. A good spotter and the power rack are your friends here. Use the rack to set the position you want to perform the Static Hold in, and then go for it.

So, how much weight should you use? Try anywhere from 10-50% more weight than you can handle with a normal range of motion.

Here's a tip: use Static Holds with a barbell in the power rack (and no wrist straps) to build both big forearms and bigger traps/neck. No spinach required.

Supersets

Two exercises performed immediately one after the other, with little to no rest between the exercises.

This technique is very effective in increasing workout intensity by increasing the training volume within a short time frame. However, they are not a particularly good technique for building strength, since you won't be able to handle the same kinds of poundage that you could do with straight sets. Especially on the second exercise when you are sucking wind.

However, supersets do have several advantages:

- **Supersets save time**

- **Supersets increase intensity** via more volume in the same time. This is called "exercise density".

- **Supersets help prevent injury** and allow you to work around injuries, since they allow you to overload muscles via volume without using max weights. The blood will flow.

There are several types of supersets you can perform. Let's take a look at each below.

Traditional

Select any two exercises for the same body part.

Here are some examples:

Body Part	Examples of Traditional Supersets
Abs	Reverse Crunches + Crunches
Back	Chins + Rows
Biceps	Preacher Curls + Barbell Curls
Chest	Presses + Flys
Delts	Presses + Laterals
Hamstrings	Lying Leg Curls + Stiff-Leg Deadlifts
Quads	Leg Extension + Leg Press
Traps	Shrugs + Upright Rows
Triceps	Dips + Pushdowns

Traditional – Pre-Exhaust

Select an isolation exercise followed by a compound exercise for the same body part.

Here are some examples:

Body Part	Examples of Pre-Exhaust Supersets
Back	Stiff-Arm Lat Pushdowns + Pulldown
Biceps	Spider Curls + Barbell Curls
Chest	Flys + Presses
Delts	Laterals + Presses
Hamstrings	Leg Curls + Stiff-Leg Deadlifts
Quads	Leg Extensions + Leg Presses
Traps	Upright Rows + Shrugs
Triceps	Pushdowns + Close-Grip Bench Press

Traditional – Post-Exhaust

Select a compound exercise followed by an isolation exercise for the same body part.

Here are some examples:

Body Part	Examples of Post-Exhaust Supersets
Back	Pulldown + Stiff-Arm Lat Pushdowns
Biceps	Barbell Curls + Spider Curls
Chest	Presses + Flys
Delts	Presses + Laterals
Hamstrings	Stiff-Leg Deadlifts + Leg Curls
Quads	Leg Presses + Leg Extensions
Traps	Shrugs + Upright Rows
Triceps	Close-Grip Bench Presses + Pushdowns

Traditional – Compound

Select two compound exercises for the same body part. Get ready for some hurt.

Here are some examples:

Body Part	Examples of Compound Supersets
Back	Bent-over Barbell Row + One-Arm Dumbbell Row
Biceps	Close-Grip Chins + Dumbbell Curls
Chest	Incline Dumbbell Press + Dips
Delts	Barbell Military Press + Arnold Press
Hamstrings	Stiff-Leg Deadlift + Reverse Lunges
Quads	Squats + Leg Press
Traps	Barbell Shrug + Dumbbell Shrug
Triceps	Close-Grip Bench Press + Dips

Traditional – Isolation

Select two isolation exercises for the same body part. Burn baby, burn.

Here are some examples:

Body Part	Examples of Isolation Supersets
Abs	Reverse Crunches + Crunches
Back	Stiff-Arm Lat Pushdowns + Dumbbell Pullovers
Biceps	Dumbbell Concentration Curls + Spider Curls
Chest	Dumbbell Flys + Cable Crossovers
Delts	Dumbbell Bent-Over Laterals + Rear Delt Machine
Hamstrings	Lying Leg Curls + Seated Leg Curls
Quads	Leg Extensions + Abductor Machine
Traps	Barbell Shrugs + Dumbbell Shrugs
Triceps	Pushdowns + Lying French Press

Antagonistic

Performing traditional supersets (two exercises for the same body part) limits the amount of weight you can use (particularly on the second exercise in the superset), due to general fatigue and lactic acid buildup. However, you can use heavier weights with antagonistic supersets because as one muscle group is working, the antagonistic muscle group is resting, and vice versa.

This technique is especially effective for improving lagging body parts, and you'll often see this used when training arms, but it's just as effective for any muscle group.

Here's a list of antagonistic muscle groups and some Antagonistic Superset examples.

Antagonistic Muscle Groups	Antagonistic Superset Examples
Chest + Back	Bench Presses + Chins
	Dips + Rows
Delts + Traps	Military Presses + Shrugs
	Arnold Presses + Upright Rows
Biceps + Triceps	Barbell Curls + Pushdowns
	Dumbbell Curls + Lying Extensions
Forearm Flexors + Extensors	Wrist Curls + Reverse Wrist Curls
Quads + Hamstrings	Squats + Stiff-Leg Deadlifts
	Leg Extensions + Lying Leg Curls
Abs + Low Back	Crunches + Hyperextensions
	Reverse Crunches + Good Mornings

Staggered

Perform a set of an exercise for a targeted muscle group immediately after every set in your normal workout. Do that for the entire workout or for a fixed number of staggered sets.

Here's what we're talking about.

Let's say you have a lagging body part (calves, rear delts, etc) or a body part that responds well to high volume training. For this example, let's say your rear delts need to be bigger in order to balance them out with your front delts, but today you are working chest. Here's what you do. After every set in your chest workout, perform a set of rear laterals. Keep doing that for the whole chest workout. In the end, you'll have performed about 12-15 sets of rear laterals using a good bit of weight. If you do this over a period of weeks, you should notice some visible improvement in the balance of your front and rear delts. Mission accomplished.

(By the way, show me someone who has over-developed rear delts, hamstrings, or calves and I'll show you how to pack on 30 pounds of muscle in 10 days. Really. Honestly.)

Weak Point Training

Inevitably, everybody is going to develop imbalances in their physique, such as asymmetry, underdevelopment of a particular body part in relation to others, etc. So, what do you do to correct that? Here are some general guidelines, followed by specific exercises that help your correct those weak points:

● Train the weak body part first in the workout.

● Train the weak body part more frequently. There are several ways to do this:

   o   Overlap the training

   o   Alternate sets for the weak body part with your regular workout

   o   Work the weak body part exclusively on its own day

   o   Increase the volume and frequency of training for the weak part

● Make sure your form is impeccable when working that body part. Many times, the weak point is related to poor exercise form.

● Make sure you are selecting the optimal exercises based on your structural limitations.

The table below lists common weak points and suggested exercises for correcting them:

Body Part	Weak Point	Suggested Exercises
Abs	Upper Abs	Incline Sit-ups, Crunches
	Lower Abs	Reverse Crunches
Back	Outer Back	Rows with a narrow grip T-Bar Rows
	Upper Back	Seated Cable Rows with a Wide-Grip (use a Lat bar) One-Arm Dumbbell Rows

Body Part	Weak Point	Suggested Exercises
	Lat Width	Wide-grip Chins and Pulldown
	Lower Lats	One-Arm Cable Rows
		Close-grip Chins, Pulldown, Bent-over Rows and Seated Rows
	Middle Back Thickness	Wide-grip Rows
		Seated Cable Rows with separate handles
		Pulldown using a close, neutral grip (palms facing each other)
	Lower Back	Deadlifts
		Hyperextensions
		Good Mornings
Biceps	Mass	Barbell Curls
		Cheat Curls
	Length & Thickness	Preacher Curls
		Incline Curls
		Arm Blaster Curls
		Prone Curls
	Peak	Concentration Curls
		Spider Curls
	Outer Thickness	Hammer Curls
		Curls with a close grip
	Inner Thickness	Curls with a wide grip
Calves	Upper Calves	Standing Calf Raises—all varieties (top half of movement, holding each rep 2-3 seconds)
	Lower Calves	Seated Calf Raises
		Calf Raises (any type) with legs slightly bent
		Partial calf raises (using

Body Part	Weak Point	Suggested Exercises
		only the bottom half of the movement)
Chest	Upper Chest	Incline Presses and Flys
		Bench Press to Neck
	Lower Chest	Dips
		Decline Presses and Flys
	Outer Chest	Dips
		Dumbbell Flys (full stretch and only the lower range of motion)
	Inner Chest	Bench Presses with narrow grip
		Presses and Flys (hold contraction at top on each rep for 2-3 seconds)
		Pec Deck with one arm
Delts	Front Delts	Military Presses
		Arnold Presses
		Upright Rows
		Front Raises
		Incline Presses and Flys
	Side Delts	Side Laterals (dumbbells/cables) starting at the sides, not in front
		Burns with heavy weight after the laterals
	Rear Delts	Start shoulder workout with rear delt exercises
		Do more sets for rear delts than side/front delts
		Bent-over laterals
		Rear Delt Machine
Forearms	Upper Forearms	Reverse Curls
		Reverse Curls on

Body Part	Weak Point	Suggested Exercises
		Preacher Bench
		Hammer Curls
		Reverse Wrist Curls
	Inner Forearms	One-Arm Wrist Curls
Glutes	Underdeveloped	Wide stance squats
		Lunges and Reverse Lunges
Hamstrings	Mass	Stiff-Leg Deadlifts
	Lack Shape	Leg Curls (all varieties), especially holding each rep for 2-3 seconds at the top
Quads	Mass	Squats
		Front Squats
		Leg Presses
	Lower Thighs	Squats, Front Squats, Hack Squats and Leg Presses (bottom half of movement only)
		Leg Extensions (hold at top for 2-3 seconds on each rep)
		Smith Machine Squats (feet out in front)
	Outer Thighs	Front and Hack Squats
		Any Squat or Leg Press with feet straight and close)
	Inner Thighs	Stiff-Leg Deadlifts
		Lunges and Side Lunges
		Any Squat or Leg Press with feet turned out and with wide stance)
		Adductor Machine
	Separation	Leg Extension

Body Part	Weak Point	Suggested Exercises
Neck	Mass	Heavy deadlifts and shrugs
Traps	Mass	Deadlifts
		Shrugs
		Upright Rows
		All rowing exercises
Triceps	Mass	Close-Grip Presses
		Weighted Dips
		Dips behind the back
		Seated French Presses
	Upper Triceps	Pushdowns (all varieties)
		Kickbacks
		(hold the contraction on each rep for 2-3 seconds)
	Lower Triceps	Weighted Dips
	Outer Head	Rope Extensions (lean forward, elbows out)

How to Work Out When You Are Injured

Inevitably, even though you consistently perform exercises with strict form in an intelligent manner, you will eventually sustain an injury. As you age, the specter of injury raises its head more often. It might be the result of chronic overuse (the archenemy of consistency), it might be due to slightly hyper-extending a joint or overstretching a tendon when performing preacher curls, calf raises, etc. It doesn't matter. You are now injured.

All is not lost.

No matter the severity of the injury, there is almost always something you can do to continue forward progress. It might not be with the body part that was injured or with body parts involved with that chain of movement, but there are several things to consider if you are injured:

- Don't ever perform an exercise that causes you pain. We're not talking muscular fatigue pain (good pain) here, but real acute pain. Find another exercise.

- Injured areas often respond well to low volume and high reps. Cut the number of sets you usually perform for that area in half and increase the reps to 15-25 on exercises that directly hit the injured area. When in doubt as to how many sets/reps to perform for an injured area, go with the rule of three: 3 sets of 15-25 reps and that's it.

- Slowly, over several weeks, try to increase your volume and lower your rep range when working the injury. Listen to your inner voice—if something doesn't feel right or pain starts increasing, stop working that area for the day. Next time, go back to your volume/rep range that you were using a couple weeks ago.

- If the injury persists or shows no sign of improvement, go to your doctor. If you have any doubt as to the severity of the injury, go to the doctor. Use common sense here.

There are specific injury prevention and recovery strategies you may want to try. In general, you should use the 1:1: Method described earlier in this book to reduce the frequency of overuse injuries. The sections below walk you through the specifics for each type of injury.

Low Back Injuries

- **Causes**: Improper form with deadlifts, squats, standing overhead presses or any type of exercise where you are bent over. Continually using very heavy weights, workout after workout, when performing the exercises mentioned above. Excessively tight hamstrings.

- **Prevention**: Strengthen your abdominals and core—always include some type of reverse crunch movement in your workouts. Stretch your hamstrings daily. Consistently perform low back exercises, such as hyperextensions or Good Mornings.

- **Workout & Recovery**: Use leg extensions (full range), leg presses and Smith Machine squats with partial range of movement when working quads. You may also be able to perform Hack Squats. Stay away from free bar squats until your back has recovered. Use chins, pulldowns, machine rows and one-arm dumbbell rows for your back work. Stay away from deadlifts or any rowing movement where you are bent over without support.

Shoulder Injuries

- **Causes**: Overuse, not cycling workout intensity, rep ranges, and exercise selection and priority. Imbalances between anterior (front) and posterior (rear) shoulder muscles. Weak rotator cuff muscles.

- **Prevention**: Rotate your lateral exercise movement workout order—in other words, if you perform front raises before rear laterals this workout, perform the rear laterals before the front raises next workout. Use cable/band adduction/abduction exercises to strengthen your rotator cuffs. When performing shoulder presses with a barbell, change the width of your grip slightly from workout to work out, and use dumbbell presses in place of the barbell frequently.

- **Workout & Recovery**: Determine which types of lateral movements (front, side, rear—dumbbells, cable, machine) you can do without any pain. Do those. Perform your shoulder presses with either the Smith

Machine or dumbbells (try a neutral grip). Group your shoulder workout with either your chest or back workout, working the shoulders last. High reps (15-25) and low volume really help with shoulder recovery.

Elbow Injuries

- **Causes**: Overuse, not changing exercises frequently enough, hyperextension.

- **Prevention**: Use the 1:1 Method when using Preacher Curls or Triceps Extensions in your workout regimen. Always warm up your elbows with high rep pushdowns and/or curls before performing arm workouts.

- **Workout & Recovery**: Lay off the preacher curls and triceps extensions. Slowly warm up with pushdowns. Perform high reps.

Knee Injuries

- **Causes**: Improper warm-up, incorrect form, weak adductor muscles.

- **Prevention**: Make sure your knee is always tracking right in line and over your foot when performing all leg movements.

- **Workout & Recovery**: Stay away from hack squats and front squats.

Neck Injuries

- **Causes**: Turning/lifting the head during any pressing or pulling movement. Improper form when shrugging.

- **Prevention**: Don't turn your head to look at the pretty girl in the gym when shrugging. Seriously, keep your head in a fixed, natural position during the set.

- **Workout & Recovery**: Perform shrugs using the Smith Machine. Use higher reps. Avoid dumbbell shrugs, heavy barbell shrugs and upright rows until the neck has recovered.

Keeping Track of Your Progress

In order to maximize your progress and the amount of muscle you can develop, you must keep accurate records of your performance. Unless you are genetically gifted toward muscle mass, there's just no way around this. Your records become a barometer of accomplishment and a roadmap for further progress.

- **You must write things down.** There is no way around this if you want to progress. You wouldn't take the longest trip of your life if you didn't have a map—would you? You need to know where you are at and where you've been, so you can determine where you need to go.

- Things you need to track: exercises, the weight used and the number of reps. It's also a good idea to include the date you did the weight/reps, so you have an indication regarding how fast you are progressing.

- Get yourself a spiral notebook, preferably one with about 300 pages so that you can record a year's worth of workouts in each notebook. Then, on each page record the date, then the exercises, weights, and reps you did.

- Use the LiftScript™ shorthand notation system (described below) to record your workout quickly.

- Circle any sets in which you achieved a personal best, **regardless of the weight used**. For example, if you reached 11 reps in the barbell curl with 100 pounds, and your previous best was 10 reps, you should circle that set.

- Once a month, you should go through your notebook and record all of the circled sets in your spreadsheet.

Wait a minute. What spreadsheet? Why do I need a spreadsheet? I don't know how to use a spreadsheet. I'll explain below. But first, let's take a look at this LiftScript™ thing.

LiftScript™

The table below summarizes the LiftScript™ notation system that will allow you to record all aspects of your workout quickly.

Symbol	Meaning	Examples
W x N	Weight x Number of reps performed (this is the basis for recording all sets)	**100x6** *100 lbs lifted for 6 reps.*
+	An indicator used to extend a set	**100x6+3F** *100 lbs lifted for 6 reps with 3 forced reps at the end.*
B	Burns	**100x6+6B** *100 lbs lifted for 6 reps with 6 burns at the end.*
F	Forced Reps	**100x8+3F** *100 lbs lifted for 8 reps with 3 forced reps at the end.*
H	Holds, Static Holds	**225x8+1H** *225 lbs lifted for 8 reps with one static hold at the end.*
N	Negatives	**100x8+3N** *100 lbs lifted for 8 reps with 3 negative reps at the end.*
P	Partial Reps (limited Range of Motion)	**120x6P** *120 lbs lifted for 6 partial range reps.*
>	Drop Sets, Strip Sets	**100x8>80x6>60x5** *100 lbs lifted for 8 reps, immediately followed (no rest) by 80 lbs for 6 reps, immediately followed by 60 lbs for 5 reps.*
/	Combination Sets (supersets, tri-sets, giant sets)	**Lying French Press/Close-Grip Press** **100x6/100x6** *100 lbs lifted in the Lying French Press for 6 reps, then 6 reps Close-Grip Presses were*

Symbol	Meaning	Examples
		performed before the set ended.
( ) x n	Multi-set shorthand notation for repeating same weight/reps over n sets	(100x8)x3 100 lbs lifted for 8 reps for 3 sets

Recording Your Progress Electronically

Once you start recording your workouts in your second notebook (you did fill up the first one, didn't you?), you'll find that it starts getting increasingly harder to remember/find/lookup just how many reps you were able to do with 195lbs on the bench press. You need to know that number—otherwise, you can throw out the whole concept of progressive resistance and go home. How can we look up this info? That's where your friend the spreadsheet comes in.

Why use a spreadsheet?

Because we're dealing primarily with numbers here (reps and pounds) that we can perform additional calculations on (such as Wilkes formulas, Power Factor, etc.), they're easy to use, update and print out, they're free (more on this below), you can use them anywhere (even on your phone) and your data can be used for decades.

Spreadsheet Options

If you already have Microsoft Excel, Microsoft Works, or another spreadsheet, you can use that for recording your progress. Otherwise, you have several free options, such as OpenOffice or Google Docs.

If you want the ultimate in a spreadsheet-based workout log, check out MuscleCALC, which works with both Microsoft Excel (Windows and Mac) and OpenOffice. MuscleCALC is already set up for you, and automatically calculates and charts your progress and indicates areas that need attention.

You can read more about MuscleCALC here:

www.runningdeersoftware.com

What You Should Record

No matter which spreadsheet software you use, you'll need to record the following info (columns) for each row on your spreadsheet:

- Name of exercise
- Weight lifted
- Number of reps performed
- The date you did it.

I recommend naming the columns in your spreadsheet: Exercise, Weight, Reps, Date

Here's an example (from MuscleCALC) showing how this would look in your spreadsheet:

MuscleCALC™			Biceps
Exercise	Weight	Reps	Date
Barbell Preacher Curls	110	10	9/5/2006
Barbell Preacher Curls	115	10	7/3/2007
Barbell Preacher Curls	120	6	8/22/2006
Barbell Preacher Curls	125	5	3/13/2007

Planning Future Workouts

If you've ever played any type of team sport, then you remember how important it is to plan your game strategy in order to maximize your chance of winning. Well guess what? It's no different when you workout.

In this case, "game time" is your workout, which means you have 3-5 games per week to get ready for. Each workout represents an investment in your time, so you better make the most of it. That means preparation and planning.

1. Before each workout, review your workout log for the last couple of workouts you did for the body parts you will be working today. This is your time to "review film" of your most recent performances.

2. Ask yourself these questions:

   ● **Should I do the same exercises again or should I pick one or more new exercises?**

   Think about the 3:1 and 1:1 Methods here.

   ● **Should I do them in the same order, or do I need to change the order?**

   Remember, *change is good.*

   ● **Did I hit a sticking point on something last time? If so, should I inject one of the Intensity Techniques into the upcoming workout?**

   Look through the list of Intensity Techniques and pick one.

   ● **For the exercises that I will be doing, what weight/rep combos should I be targeting?**

   You need your workout log and playbook to answer this. In this case, your playbook is the spreadsheet that you built to record your best efforts. (If you are using the MuscleCALC spreadsheet, it will help generate your playbook for you.)

If you don't take the time to prepare and plan your upcoming workout, you're simply relying on genetics and memory to get you through. That may work for awhile, but eventually you're gonna get cut from the team—in this case, your body will stop growing muscle and you'll join the legions of lemmings simply going through the motions of working out, with no return on your investment. Invest the time and effort and build up the Bank of You.

And finally, remember—when seeking success, look first to yourself.

Cardio

Let's get this out of the way: **Cardiovascular exercise is a catabolic process. It eats away muscle**. So, if your goal is to build as much muscle as possible, you shouldn't do it, should you? Well, let's talk about that.

Why do people do cardio in the first place? There's really only two answers—either they think they need to lose body fat or they do it to increase athleticism (to feel and be fit).

Cardio isn't the best way to reduce body fat—having slabs of muscle hanging off your body is. Coupled with a proper diet, of course. When you take an aerobics class, or schlep on over to the stationary bike, you are engaging in an activity that temporarily increases your metabolism, thus burning calories at a faster rate than you normally would. Notice the word 'temporary'. If that's all you do—just cardio—you are living a grand illusion. However, if you emphasize weight training as I've discussed above, you'll create a permanent increase in your basal metabolic rate—you'll burn more calories, all the time, like a steam locomotive with an endless supply of coal. More muscle + strict diet = low body fat.

Now, if you are doing cardio to increase athleticism, what you are really doing is increasing your VO2Max—your ability to efficiently use oxygen during activity. Any activity—even weight training. That's a good thing.

So, the big questions surrounding cardio are how often should I do it (if at all), how long should I do it, when should I do it, and what type of cardio is best. In essence, those are questions of frequency, duration, timing, and selection—all similar questions that we answered for weight training. Here, the answers are different.

The Two Types of Cardio

You can do cardio two ways—long duration at low intensity (steady state), or shorter duration at high intensity. You measure intensity by calculating your Target Heart Rate Range and making sure your heart rate (beats per minute = bpm) stays within that range:

- Target Heart Rate Range (low intensity) = (220 – Your Age) x 60%-75%

- Target Heart Rate Range (high intensity) = (220- Your Age) x 80%-90%

For example, if you are 30 years old and weigh 180lbs, your low intensity THR is 114-142bpm and your high-intensity THR is 152-171bpm.

So, there are two basic types of cardio—which should you do?

Let's think about it this way. Look at your average marathon runner. You have someone who runs at low intensity for very long durations. Typically, their bodies are skinny, with relatively little muscle. Now, think about the 100m sprinter who runs at high intensity for very short duration. Their bodies can exhibit significant muscle mass along with low body fat. However, their cardiovascular endurance does not match up to the marathoner.

- **You should alternate between both types of cardio, from cardio workout to cardio workout.** This will diversify your cardiovascular profile, providing you with the benefits of both, prevent boredom (I hope), and keep your body responding.

- **A particularly effective way to perform high-intensity cardio is by using interval training**, alternating periods of low-intensity with high-intensity during the cardio session. I like to use the stationary bike for 20-30 minutes of interval training where I pedal for 80rpm for 15-30 seconds, and the remainder of each minute for 100rpm. This is High-Intensity Interval Training (HIIT).

How Often Should I Do Cardio?

Keep the frequency of cardio training to a minimum, based on body type and your current level of fitness.

- **Ectomorphs (those naturally skinny): 2-3 times per week using only high-intensity , low duration.**

- **Endomorphs (if you tend to hold fat) and Mesomorphs (if you are naturally muscular): 3-5 times per week, alternating between high and low intensity cardio sessions.**

- **Do as few sessions as possible per week that allows you to gain the benefits of your approach**. If you have a lot of fat to get rid of, do more sessions per week.

How Long Should I Do Cardio?

The level of intensity you select will dictate the optimal duration of your cardio session.

- **Low Intensity Cardio: 30-45 minutes**

- **High Intensity Cardio: 15-30 minutes**

When Should I Do My Cardio?

The timing of your cardio depends largely on your lifestyle and schedule. As your options become limited, so too can the effectiveness of the results.

- **Optimally, in the morning, upon rising**. This will produce the greatest fat-burning results.

- **Ideally, on days you don't train with weights**. For those unemployed, independently wealthy, or needing balance in their lives. If you have the time, low intensity is the way to go here.

- **Otherwise, after your weight training sessions**. The option for the rest of us, with families, obligations, and a life.

I perform my cardio three times per week, after my weight training sessions, alternating between low and high intensity techniques. I use weight training and diet as the base for building muscle and staying lean, while using cardio to improve heart function and burn a little more calories, as needed.

Finally, it really doesn't matter if you like to do your cardio with the stationary bike, elliptical trainer, treadmill, Step Mill, or running around outside. Just make sure you have a plan, track your heart rate, and be consistent. Like Lance said, it's not about the equipment—it's the heart, desire, and execution.

A Word about Your Diet

You could write a whole book about how to construct an optimal diet for maximizing muscle building while maintaining a lean physique. But here, we're sticking primarily to the weightlifting stuff. However, since diet is so very important to your success in building quality, lean muscle, we don't want to leave you hanging—so, follow these dietary guidelines to accelerate your muscle building progress.

- **Protein is king.** It's how your body builds muscle. Most people don't eat enough protein to make really significant muscle gains. Medical sources will tell you that about 0.8 grams of protein per pound of body weight is a good amount. That might work for Clark Kent, but not for Superman. Bodybuilding sources will tell you that anywhere from 1-2 grams per pound of body weight is a good target. Just cut to the chase and always eat 2 grams per pound of body weight and watch the magic happen. Your protein intake should equate to 40-50% of your total calories for the day.

- Since you'll need high levels of low-fat protein sources, **plan on drinking half of your daily protein requirements in the form of whey/casein powdered drinks**. You simply won't be able to get two grams of protein per pound of body weight without doing this.

- **As soon as you get up, drink a whey-based protein drink.** This quick-release protein will get into your blood stream rapidly.

- **Most people eat too many carbs, or the wrong types of carbs.** You want to eat low glycemic, slow-burning carbs like oatmeal with your first meal of the day, vegetables for your carb source for all the other meals, except your post-workout meal.

- **Your post workout meal is special.** By post-workout, we mean from 1-60 minutes after you stop working out. That's your window of opportunity, when your body can assimilate protein and carbs much more efficiently than at any other period. Therefore, you want to **drink a quick-acting whey protein immediately after you stop working out** (something with at least 30 grams protein), and something that has simple carbs (at least as many, if not more carbs as grams of protein). A perfect example is one of those post-workout drinks that has roughly 30 grams protein and 50 grams of carbs. Then, go home and eat a good food-based meal with lean protein and carbs (chicken/turkey and potato).

● **Drink at least one gallon of water a day.** Two gallons if you are trying to get leaner.

● **Take a casein-based protein drink right before you go to bed.** This slow-digesting protein will be like hooking a protein-based IV drip up to you for the next 3-4 hours that you sleep. Couple that with some good REM sleep, and that's a recipe for some serious recovery and growth.

● **Don't combine a high-carb meal with a high-fat meal.** That's a deadly combination. High-protein/high-carb/low-fat is ok, and so is high-protein/low-carb/low-fat. Just don't do low-protein/high-carb/high-fat. In case you haven't noticed, just about all fast-food restaurants are centered around serving the deadly combo. Stay away— except for one exception (see below).

● If you are trying to flush a lot of water out of your body (let's say you are going to hit the beach tomorrow), then double your water intake, ramp up the Vitamin C (use the 500mg chewable tablets), and cut out the complex carbs. This combo will act as a natural diuretic and help to rid your body of subcutaneous water.

Recommended Foods

Try to eat exclusively from this recommended list of foods, in order to optimize your muscle building progress. Of course, it's ok for your sanity (and your metabolism) to stray from this list *only on limited or planned occasions.*

Protein

- Chicken Breast (no skin)
- Turkey (white meat)
- Fish (tuna, salmon, cod, tilapia, snapper)
- Beef (90% or leaner; filet, sirloin, round, flank)
- Eggs (limit the yolks; unlimited whites)
- Cottage cheese (good natural source of casein protein)

Vegetables (Fibrous Carbs)

- Asparagus, broccoli, Brussels sprouts, cabbage, carrots, cauliflower, celery, cucumbers, egg plant, green beans, lettuce (all types), mushrooms, okra, onions, peppers (all types), spinach, squash (summer only), tomatoes, zucchini

Starchy Carbs

- Acorn squash, barley, beans (black, lima, kidney, red), black-eyed peas, corn, cream of rice, Ezekiel bread, oatmeal, popcorn (air-popped, unsalted), potatoes (all types), rice (brown or long-grain), Wasa crackers

Fruits

- Apples, bananas (limit these), blueberries, cantaloupe, grapefruit, oranges, peaches, pears, pineapple, raspberries, strawberries

Healthy Fats

- Almonds, almond butter, cashew butter, heavy whipping cream, peanut butter, walnuts

- Oils (flaxseed, olive, safflower, sunflower)

Beverages

- Water, tea, coffee

Condiments

- Garlic, lemon juice, lime juice, mustard, seasonings (dried), vinegar

Food	Serving Size	Cal	Protein	Carbs	Fat
Proteins					
Chicken/Turkey Breast (skinless)	3 oz	135	25	0	3
Salmon	3 oz	175	19	0	11
Tilapia/Cod	3 oz	80	17	0	1
Tuna/Snapper	3 oz	100	22	0	1
Filet, Sirloin, Round, Flank Steak	3 oz	180	25	0	7
Egg	1 large	90	6	1	7
Egg White	1 large	36	6	0	0
Cottage Cheese	1 cup	123	25	3	1
Vegetables (Fibrous Carbs)					
Asparagus, Brussels sprouts, green beans, kale, okra, tomatoes	1 cup	35	2	7	0
Broccoli, cauliflower, celery, peppers	1cup	25	2	4	0
Cabbage, cucumbers, egg plant, summer squash, zucchini	1 cup	20	1	4	0
Lettuce, spinach	1 cup	10	1	1	0
Carrots	1 cup	55	1	13	0
Onions	1 cup	90	3	21	0
Mushrooms	1 cup	42	3	8	0
Starchy Carbs					
Acorn squash	1 cup	56	1	15	0
Barley, rice (cooked)	1 cup	200	5	44	1
Beans	1 cup	220	15	40	1
Black-eyed peas	1 cup	32	2	7	0
Corn	1 cup	150	6	36	1
Cream of rice	¼ cup	170	3	36	0
Ezekiel bread	1 slice	80	4	14	1
Oatmeal	½ cup	150	5	27	3
Popcorn (air-popped, plain)	1 cup	20	1	5	0
Potatoes	1 medium	220	5	51	0
Fruits					

Food	Serving Size	Cal	Protein	Carbs	Fat
Apples, grapefruit	1 medium	80	0	20	0
Banana, pear	1 medium	105	1	25	0
Blueberries	Handful	40	0	10	0
Cantaloupe	1 cup	56	1	13	0
Oranges	1 medium	62	1	15	0
Peaches	1 medium	42	1	11	0
Pineapple	1 cup	80	1	19	0
Raspberries	1 cup	60	1	14	2
Strawberries	1 cup	44	1	10	0
Healthy Fats					
Almonds	1 oz (approx 24)	165	6	6	14
Almond butter, cashew butter, peanut butter	1 Tbsp	100	3	3	9
Oils (canola, flaxseed, olive)	1 Tbsp	120	0	0	14

The Workouts

This section presents battle-tested workouts designed to keep your muscle building progress moving forward. Think of them as Shock and Awe for your body. Good luck. This is gonna hurt.

You'll see the following abbreviations used throughout the workouts:

Abbreviation	Full Name
BB	Barbell
DB	Dumbbell
Smith	Smith Machine

Some notes about the workouts:

- **Each section starts with Foundation workouts.** These workouts use primarily Key Exercises and should form the basis for your own workouts. These are the workouts you'll come back to time and time again. Subsequent workouts emphasize various intensity techniques. Use them to force muscle growth to continue.

- Unless otherwise noted, increase your weights each set using the standard half-pyramid technique.

- If specific grip or stance widths are required or particular ranges of motion should be used they are noted—otherwise use your normal grip/stance and a full range of motion.

- Each workout is prefaced with some narrative to let you know what to expect and what you should feel.

- Why do the workouts have names? Because after you do them, you'll remember them by name. Curse them by name. Maybe even come to love them by name. Plus, it's just plain interesting to give them names, instead of tossing them out there as nameless entities. Each workout has a story that you will learn and many may become etched in your consciousness forever.

- Why do some body parts have a lot of workouts listed and others not as many? Because these aren't cookie-cutter workouts—they came from personal log books of the most effective workouts performed by the supermen over the past 20 years.

Run the Gauntlet

See if you can complete every workout in the book. I dare you.

Abs

Ab workouts are all about crunches and various twisting exercises for your core. You can largely forget about sit-ups, unless you are really interested in strengthening your psoas and illiapsoas muscles and not your rectus abdominus (e.g., six-pack). Performing primarily reverse crunches will hit your entire abdominal wall and help eliminate the common lower ab weakness.

Foundation I

Exercise	Sets (6)	Reps
Reverse Crunches	4	To failure
Crunches	2	To failure

Foundation II

Exercise	Sets (8)	Reps
Reverse Crunches	4	To failure
Broomstick Twists	2	25-100
Crunches	2	To failure

Crunch Time

Here's one of the most effective ab routines you can do. This one is based around the trunk moving towards your pelvis. Perform the exercises as a tri-set.

Exercise	Sets (1-5 tri-sets)	Reps
Crunches	1-5	To failure
Lying Twists	1-5	To failure
Twisting Crunches	1-5	To failure

Put It in Reverse

Another effective ab routine—this one concentrating on bringing the pelvis towards the chest and really activating the lower abs. Perform the reverse crunches on a flat or incline surface, or hanging, depending on your strength level.

Exercise	Sets (6)	Reps
Reverse Crunches	6	25

Chest

I'm going to start the chest workout section with workouts that emphasize incline pressing movements for the upper chest, since that's where most people have deficiencies. I also think optimal chest workouts are comprised of predominantly pressing movements with some fly movements included for complete pectoral kinetics. It's also a good idea to alternate pressing exercises with fly exercises, since this helps you use maximal weights in both types of movements, giving you a little mental rest between the presses.

Foundation I

Exercise	Sets (12)	Reps
Incline Barbell or Dumbbell Bench Press	4	12, 10, 8, 6
Incline or Flat Dumbbell Fly	4	10-12 reps
Barbell Bench Press	4	6-8 reps

Foundation II

Exercise	Sets (12)	Reps
Barbell Bench Press	4	12, 10, 8, 6
Incline Dumbbell Fly	4	10-12 reps
Dips	4	To failure

Getting Stronger

Here we are modifying the Foundation I workout rep range to build more strength and power.

Exercise	Sets (12)	Reps
Incline Bench Press	5	8, 4, 3, 3 negatives, 5
Flat Dumbbell Fly	3	8, 8, 8
Barbell Bench Press	4	8, 4, 2, 4

With a Little Help from My Friend

All upper chest work. You can use it. In this case, the Smith Machine is your friend—or is he?

Exercise	Sets (15)	Reps
Smith Machine Incline Press	6	10, 8, 6, 5, 5, 6
Incline Dumbbell Fly	3	6-8
Smith Bench Press (to neck)	6	6

Mr. Smith Goes to Hell

This workout turns the nice, easy Smith Machine into an anabolic-inducing monster with bite at the end.

Exercise	Sets (15)	Reps
Smith Incline Press (30°)	6	15, 12, 10, 8, 4, 6
Smith Incline Press (50°)	3	6, 6, 6
Dumbbell Fly (20°)	3	10, 10, 10
Dips	3	6, 6, 6

Dumbbells on My Mind

After letting the Smith Machine guide you, you guide the dumbbells in the last half of this workout.

Exercise	Sets (14)	Reps
Smith Machine Incline Press	6	20, 8, 8, 6, 6, 6
Incline or Flat Dumbbell Fly	4	20, 15, 10, 10
Dumbbell Press	4	2, 3, 5, 25

Press On

This one is all pressing, which you'll be after you are done. Your upper chest is gonna get fried.

Exercise	Sets (12)	Reps
Incline Bench Press	5	12, 6, 4, 4, 12
Barbell Bench Press	3	6, 4, 15
Smith Machine Incline Press	4	6, 6, 10, 12

Go Big or Go Home

After a proper warm-up, go right into a traditional, time-tested strength and power groove of 5x5, followed by another staple of 6x6. Then, a quick blood rushing finish at the end. Take lots of rest for the first nine workout sets of this one. You want big weights here.

Exercise	Sets (14)	Reps
Incline Barbell Press	3	Warm up sets
Incline Barbell Press	5	5, 5, 5, 5, 5
Barbell Bench Press	4	6, 6, 6, 6
Pec Dec	1	12
Dumbbell Pullover	1	10

Guillotine

Performing presses to the neck is dangerous (less so on the Smith Machine) but highly effective for the upper pecs. If you survive the first exercise, you get seven more sets of presses as your reward.

Exercise	Sets (17)	Reps
Smith Bench Press (to neck)	6	15, 8, 4, 4, 10, 10
Incline Dumbbell Press	4	6, 6, 6, 15
Incline Barbell Press	3	6, 6, 4
Incline Dumbbell Fly	4	8, 4, 4, 20

Nothing Fancy I

Nothing fancy here—just pure volume and variety.

Exercise	Sets (18)	Reps
Incline Barbell Press	6	12, 10, 10, 8, 6, 4
Barbell Bench Press	4	8, 8, 8, 8
Dips	4	8, 8, 8, 8
Flat Dumbbell Fly	3	6, 6, 6
Dumbbell Pullover	1	12

Basic Variety I

Start with some basics, and then go for variety. This will get your chest from all angles.

Exercise	Sets (18)	Reps
Incline Barbell Press	7	10, 10, 10, 6, 6, 6, 8
Flat Dumbbell Press	3	12, 10, 8
Flat Dumbbell Fly	2	6, 6
Dips	2	to failure
Dumbbell Pullover	2	10, 10
Cable Crossover	2	8, 8

Exhaustion

The finish to this workout has you performing a traditional pre-exhaust combination superset. Sometimes that's all it takes to get the adaptation process started or keep it rolling on.

Exercise	Sets (11)	Reps
Incline Dumbbell Press	6	15, 12, 10, 8, 6, 4
Barbell Bench Press	3	4, 8, 12
Decline Dumbbell Fly + Press	2	8+8, 8+8

End of Day

Looks typical, but just when you think you're done, I need you to perform a 1RM effort on the bench press with a drop-set. Huh? Yeah, that's the end of your workout.

Exercise	Sets (11)	Reps
Incline Dumbbell Press	6	15, 12, 10, 8, 8, 8
Dumbbell Fly	3	20, 15, 12 (same weight)
Barbell Bench Press	2	10, 1>8

Ascent

This workout hits your upper pecs hard and fast, and then you get to lie down and find out how much mental toughness you have. Choose your weights wisely on that last exercise.

Exercise	Sets (10)	Reps
Incline Barbell Press	5	15, 12, 10, 8, 6
Incline Dumbbell Press	2	10, 8
Dumbbell Fly	3	15, 25, 30 (same weight)

Confusion

A lot happens in this workout. The first half has you performing the entire spectrum of rep ranges on the Smith Machine. Believe me, you'll appreciate the guidance. Then, a nice little break with the flys, ending with some ass-heavy benching with whatever you've got left. You do have something left, don't you?

Exercise	Sets (12)	Reps
Smith Machine Incline Press	6	15, 12, 10, 4, 4, 20
Incline Dumbbell Fly	3	10,10, 10 (same weight)
Barbell Bench Press	3	5, 5, 5 (same weight)

Pump Up the Volume: Upper Chest Edition

This time it's lot's of sets, but you start with the upper chest first.

Exercise	Sets (19)	Reps
Incline Bench Press	5	10,6-8, 6-8, 4, 6-8
Barbell Bench Press	5	10, 6-8, 4, 2, 6
Dips	3	12, 10, 8
Flat Dumbbell Fly	3	6-8
Dumbbell Pullover	3	10-12

Pump Up the Volume: Chest Edition

Volume is the basis for this workout—lot's more sets than you should typically perform. Use it sparingly and get ready for the hurt.

Exercise	Sets (23)	Reps
Barbell Bench Press	5	12, 10, 8, 6, 4
Incline Bench Press	5	10, 8, 6, 6, 4-6
Decline Dumbbell Press	5	6-8
Flat Dumbbell Fly	3	6-8
Dumbbell Pullover	3	15
Cable Crossover	2	15

Angular Attraction

This workout has lots of volume and variety. It will hit your chest from every angle making for a very symmetrical, attractive look.

Exercise	Sets (18)	Reps
Barbell Bench Press	5	12, 8, 5, 3, 8
Incline Bench Press	4	12, 8, 5, 3
Flat Dumbbell Fly	3	10, 10, 8
Dips	3	10, 10, 10
Dumbbell Pullover	3	12, 12, 12

Keep On Rollin'

Lots of volume here, with alternating press and fly movements to get you through.

Exercise	Sets (19)	Reps
Barbell Bench Press	8	15, 12, 10, 6, 4, 2, 15, 15
Flat Dumbbell Fly	4	15, 5, 5, 15
Incline Bench Press	4	10, 6, 6, 6
Cable Crossover	3	12, 6, 20

Deception

This one looks pretty standard. Start off with the barbell, go to the Smith machine, then finish with pullovers. But watch out for that 20 rep set in there. Then, show me how much you have left on the Smith machine.

Exercise	Sets (15)	Reps
Barbell Bench Press	9	12, 8, 6, 4, 2, 2, 4, 6, 20
Smith Machine Incline Press	3	8, 8, 8
Dumbbell Pullover	3	15, 10, 8

Defining Moment

Very similar to the workout above, except a little more balanced and no surprise 20 rep set. Here the Pec Dec will be your defining moment.

Exercise	Sets (13)	Reps
Barbell Bench Press	7	12, 8, 6, 6, 6, 12, 12
Smith Machine Incline Press	5	6, 6, 6, 6, 12
Pec Dec	1	5, followed by 2 drops

Defining Moment II

Another high volume workout, with alternating press and fly movements, with the emphasis on pressing. Check out that last set. That's supposed to be done as heavy as possible. Really.

Exercise	Sets (18)	Reps
Barbell Bench Press	8	15, 8, 4, 4, 6, 6, 6, 8
Dumbbell Fly (flat)	4	10, 8, 10, 20
Incline Barbell Press	5	10, 3, 3, 3, 10
Cable Crossover	1	25

Little Bit Of Everything

After starting with some basic pressing, we go for maximum variety while confusing your chest with fly and pressing movements, drastic rep range variations, and a test of maximum will and effort for the final three sets.

Exercise	Sets (16)	Reps
Barbell Bench Press	7	20, 10, 6, 6, 3, 6, 6
Incline Dumbbell Fly	4	10, 6, 6, 15
Incline Barbell Press	2	5, 5
Pec Dec	1	15
Cable Crossover	1	15
Dumbbell Pullover	1	15

Around the World in 80 Reps

Bill Pearl's famous Around the World dumbbell workout. Don't forget to reverse direction once you get half the reps completed for each set of Around the Worlds. This exercise really taxes your chest, anterior delts and biceps. Just make sure you warm up properly and don't worry about really heavy weights on this one—just concentrate on form and motion. You can do this on a flat bench or incline for variation.

Exercise	Sets (10)	Reps
Dumbbell Around the World	4	20
Barbell Bench Press	6	6

Jason and the Pectorals

This workout is named in honor of my friend Jason. Years ago, he came into the gym, said "I only have 10 minutes to work my chest. Give me something that will really work it." Here's the result. Three quick warm-up sets, followed by one continuous drop-set of barbell bench presses (flat or incline) using 10lb weights piled out to the ends of the bar.

Exercise	Sets (1)	Reps
Barbell Bench Press (flat or incline)	1 continuous drop-set	To failure

Reverse Logic

An unusual start with the Pec Dec. And check out those high reps tacked onto the end of each series.

Exercise	Sets (19)	Reps
Pec Dec	4	15, 12, 10, 25
Barbell Bench Press	5	10, 8, 4, 4, 15
Incline Dumbbell Fly	5	15, 12, 6, 4, 15
Incline Barbell Press	5	10, 5, 5, 5, 10

Good Luck

This one has everything—volume, variety, failure and supersets. Here failure is success.

Exercise	Sets (19)	Reps
Barbell Bench press	9	10, 10, 8, 3, 3, 3, 6, 6, 6
Incline Dumbbell Press	3	8, 6, 6
Incline Dumbbell Fly	3	6, 6, 6
Dips	2	To failure
Cable Crossover/DB Pullover	2	6/10, 6/10

More Damn Good Luck

This one starts out with plenty of basic pressing, and then kills you with a combination superset. If you are still able to move your pecs, then either the Dips or the last two sets of Pec Dec will get you.

Exercise	Sets (19)	Reps
Barbell Bench Press	9	15, 10, 10, 8, 4, 4, 4, 6, 6
Incline Dumbbell Fly/Press	4	6/6, 6/6, 6/6, 6/6
Dips	3	6, 6, 6
Pec Dec	3	8, 15, 30

Unleash Hell

A pretty standard chest workout, except this time you're going for a one-rep max effort. Take it easy until you get there. Then, unleash hell. And keep unleashing it for the rest of the workout.

Exercise	Sets (12)	Reps
Barbell Bench Press	7	20, 10, 10, 3, 3, 1, 8
Dumbbell Fly	3	25, 20, 15
Incline Dumbbell Press	2	10, 10

All Bases Covered

Here you will perform across the entire rep range spectrum, finishing with a test of character.

Exercise	Sets (12)	Reps
Barbell Bench Press	6	20, 12, 10, 8, 5, 2
Smith Machine Incline Press	4	10, 10, 4, 8
Dips	2	To failure

Nothin' but Supersets

Now we really get going with some supersets. An entire workout of nothing but supersets. Burn baby, burn. This workout would go great after a previous heavy lifting session.

Exercise	Sets (7)	Reps
Flat Dumbbell Press/Fly	4	30/15, 20/10, 10/10, 8/8
Incline Dumbbell Press/Fly	3	20/10, 12/10, 8/10

Taste of Germany

This workout incorporates a little taste of German Volume Training on the second exercise.

Exercise	Sets (14)	Reps
Barbell Bench Press	5	15, 12, 10, 6, 6
Incline Dumbbell Press	7	10, 10, 10, 10, 10, 10, 10
Cable Crossover	2	12, 10

Range Rover

The purpose here is to work on handling some very heavy weights in the top half range of the barbell bench press. Do this workout in a power rack.

Exercise	Sets (13)	Reps
Bench Press (full range)	5	15, 10, 6, 6, 6
Bench Press (top half range)	4	5, 5, 5, 5
Bench Press (full range)	1	12
Incline Dumbbell Press	3	12, 10, 8

Crossing Over

The only unusual thing here is that you'll perform the cable crossovers seated, with your chest against the pad of the bench. No cheating that way and you might feel something new.

Exercise	Sets (12)	Reps
Barbell Bench Press	6	15,, 10, 8, 6, 4, 12
Cable Crossover (seated)	3	10, 10, 10
Incline Dumbbell Press	3	6, 6, 6

Back

"Row, row, row your back." Chins and rows are the bedrock of back exercise workouts. Of course, you can't ignore deadlifts either. But for sheer width and thickness, nothing beats chins and rows. The following workouts will take you across a vast landscape of chin/pulldown and rowing combinations that will make anyone's back wider and thicker.

Foundation I

Exercise	Sets (12)	Reps
Chins (to the front)	3	To failure
Bent-over Barbell Row	3	6-12
Pulldown (to rear)	3	8-12
One-Arm Dumbbell Row	3	8-12

Foundation II

Exercise	Sets (16)	Reps
Bent-over Barbell Row	4	6-12
Chins (to front)	4	6-12
T-Bar Row	4	6-10
Pulldown (to rear)	4	8-12

Negative Attitude

A really good way to increase chinning strength is to perform negatives on the chin bar. Couple this with added resistance and muscular failure and you have a recipe for some true latissimus destruction. This is a very tough workout all the way around.

Exercise	Sets (15)	Reps
Chins (to front)	3	10+2 negatives, 8+2 negatives, 6+2 negatives
T-Bar Row	3	8, 4, 8
Pulldown (to front)	3	5
Seated Cable Row	3	10, 10, 5
Pulldown (close-grip)	3	6-8, 6-8, 4

Déjà vu

This one ends how it started. Lucky you. In between are heavy rows and pulldowns.

Exercise	Sets (15)	Reps
Chins (to front)	5	To failure
T-Bar Row	6	6, 6, 6, 6, 6, 6
Pulldown (to rear)	3	8, 8, 8
Chins (to front)	1	To failure

Power Up

Every once in awhile it's a good idea to incorporate a heavy overload movement with a weight you might not be able to handle through a full range of motion. In this case, we're talking about partial deadlifts in the power rack for building thick spinal erectors and a thickened back.

Exercise	Sets (15)	Reps
Chins (to front)	3	To failure
Bent-over Barbell Row	5	8, 8, 4, 4, 4
Pulldown (neutral grip)	3	10, 6, 6
Partial Deadlift (power rack)	4	6, 6, 6, 6

Stay the Course

Here is a relatively low-volume back workout that has you staying within 6-8 reps throughout. A pure mass builder. Make sure you strap on some weight for the chins if you need it.

Exercise	Sets (10)	Reps
Chins (to front)	4	8, 8, 8, 8
One-Arm Dumbbell Row	3	8, 8, 8
Pulldown (neutral grip)	3	6, 6, 6

Bombastic

Simple, basic, and tough. Dave Draper would be proud.

Exercise	Sets (12)	Reps
Chins (to front)	4	To failure
Reverse-Grip Pulldown	4	8, 8, 8, 8
Bentover Barbell Row	4	6, 6, 6, 6

No Rows Allowed

As the name implies, this workout has no rowing movements involved. Use this high-volume workout when you want to concentrate on widening those lats.

Exercise	Sets (17)	Reps
Chins (to front)	4	To failure
Pulldown (to rear)	5	8, 8, 8, 15, 15
Pulldown (neutral grip)	5	8, 8, 8, 15, 15
Dumbbell Pullover	3	6, 6, 6

Wide Load

This high-volume workout has several special characteristics. 50 reps on the chins to start. Heavy rows which follow. Grip changes. And a building crescendo of reps to blow your back up like a balloon.

Exercise	Sets (16)	Reps
Chins (to rear)	5	10, 10, 10, 10, 10
Bentover Barbell Row	5	6, 6, 6, 6, 6
Pulldown (neutral grip)	4	10, 5, 5, 15
Pulldown (wide, to front)	2	20, 20

My Three Grips

You'll use all three types of grips on this workout—pronated, supinated, and neutral.

Exercise	Sets (16)	Reps
Chins (to front)	8	10, 10, 10, 10, 10, 10, 10, 10
One-Arm Dumbbell Row	3	8, 8, 8
Reverse-Grip Pulldown	3	15, 12, 8
Hyperextension	2	15, 15

'100'

One hundred reps of chins in as few sets as possible. Don't sacrifice form. If somehow, you can get 100 reps in five sets or less, then strap on the dipping belt and some plates and start again.

Exercise	Sets (?)	Reps
Chins (any type)	As few as possible	100 total reps in as few sets as possible

Viking Ship

Viking ships were heavy, massive structures of wood. The men that rowed these ships forged themselves in the bowels of the rowmen's seats. Here, you get to row one for the last half of the workout.

Exercise	Sets (13)	Reps
Chins (to front)	4	To failure
Reverse-Grip Pulldown	3	15, 12, 10
Seated Cable Row	6	6, 6, 6, 6, 6, 6

Viking Ship: Extended Tour

After the Viking ships landed on the shores of their foes, they set fire to their boats, ensuring no return without victory. Here, after warming up with chins, and readying yourself with heavy pulldowns, you'll row to shore and see what kind of man you will become with the ultimate test of strength—deadlifts. Except, I'll take pity on your first voyage and let you do them on the Smith Machine.

Exercise	Sets (12)	Reps
Chins	3	To failure
Reverse-Grip Pulldown	3	6, 6, 6
Seated Cable Row	3	5, 5, 5
Smith Machine Deadlift	3	6, 6, 6

Crucifixion

If you thought the '100' workout was tough—try this one. You may actually end up doing more than 100 total reps of chins here, since you need to do ten sets. Plus, you get a bonus three sets of rows for good measure.

Exercise	Sets (13)	Reps
Chins (to rear)	10	As many as possible
Seated Cable Row	3	10, 10, 10

Neutralized

This workout uses a neutral grip throughout, giving you a nice overload with that grip.

Exercise	Sets (12)	Reps
Pulldown (neutral grip)	7	10, 10, 10, 10, 10, 10, 10
T-Bar Row	5	8, 8, 8, 8, 8

Rowmageddon

This workout primarily consists of rowing movements. The pulldowns will get your lats warmed up and full of blood, then it's off on a tour of rowing movements. Any rowing movement where you are bent-over makes it tough to breath, especially with heavy weight. Here you get two of these movements, but we do give you a little break with the cable in between.

Exercise	Sets (13)	Reps
Pulldown (to front)	4	10, 10, 8, 8
T-Bar Row	3	6-8
Seated Cable Row	3	10, 10, 10
Bent-over Barbell Row	3	4-6

Good Night

You will be ready to say goodbye to this workout after those last three sets of Good Mornings. Make sure that you keep increasing the amount of resistance you are holding while doing that exercise.

Exercise	Sets (13)	Reps
Pulldown (to front)	4	12, 10, 10, 10
Reverse-Grip Pulldown	3	8, 8, 8
Seated Cable Row	3	12, 6, 6
Good Mornings	3	20, 12, 10

Neutral Zone

Here's a high-volume workout where you'll spend the latter half with your hands in the neutral position. Really try to pull those elbows back as far as possible on each of those exercises.

Exercise	Sets (15)	Reps
Pulldown (to front)	5	15, 12, 10, 8, 4
Pulldown (neutral grip)	2	15, 15
T-Bar Row	4	6, 6, 6, 6
Seated Cable Row	4	12, 12, 12, 12

Handle of the Earth

Half of this workout will have you doing heavy pulldowns with various grips. The last two sets of dumbbell rows need to be performed with some of the heaviest dumbbells you've ever handled.

Exercise	Sets (10)	Reps
Reverse-Grip Pulldown	5	15, 10, 6, 6, 6
Pulldown (neutral grip)	3	12, 6, 6
One-Arm Dumbbell Row	2	3, 3

Tough Enough

Chins are a tough enough movement themselves. Performing them after your lats are starting to fatigue takes them to another level of intensity. Use your body weight on them and go to complete failure.

Exercise	Sets (12)	Reps
Reverse-Grip Pulldown	7	15, 12, 10, 8, 6, 6, 4
Chins (to rear)	3	to failure
One-Arm Dumbbell Row	2	6, 6

Gasping for Air

Again, here we are with chins placed after your lats have been pre-fatigued by the pulldowns. This time, you'll be gasping for air as you attempt to get your three sets of ten on the bent-over rows.

Exercise	Sets (12)	Reps
Pulldown (neutral grip)	3	15, 10, 8
Reverse-Grip Pulldown	3	8, 8, 8
Chins (any type)	3	to failure
Bent-over Barbell Row	3	10, 10, 10

Holy Rowing Hell!

This workout starts with rows and continues with rows until the last three sets, finishing with a high rep set to force as much blood as possible into your already swollen lats.

Exercise	Sets (14)	Reps
Bent-over BB Row	8	12, 8, 8, 8, 8, 6, 6, 12
Seated Cable Row	3	8, 6, 10
Reverse-Grip Pulldown	2	8, 8
Pulldown (to front)	1	20

Gasping for Air II

You'll be bent-over for the first nine sets of this workout. Take your time to catch your breath between sets—we don't want you to experience the deleterious effects of the Valsalva maneuver here.

Exercise	Sets (12)	Reps
Bent-over BB Row	6	12, 10, 10, 6, 6, 6
T-Bar Row	3	15, 15, 10
Reverse-Grip Pulldown	2	6, 6
Pulldown (to rear)	1	15

T-Bar Nation

This workout gives you a nice tour of the landscape of rep ranges on the T-Bar Row.

Exercise	Sets (14)	Reps
T-Bar Row	5	10, 10, 8, 4, 20
Chins (to front)	4	6, 6, 6, 6
Pulldown (neutral grip)	4	6, 6, 6, 20

More T-Bar Nation

Since you liked the T-Bar Nation so much, we've extended the tour with some follow-up deadlifts, pulldowns, and chins for a complete experience.

Exercise	Sets (16)	Reps
T-Bar Row	5	15, 10, 8, 8, 20
Deadlift	3	12, 10, 4
Pulldown (neutral grip)	3	10, 4, 6
Pulldown (wide, to front)	3	6, 6, 6
Chins (to front)	2	6, 6

Burning Lats

This is a fairly high-rep workout throughout. Most individuals are not used to performing 20 reps on a set of pulldowns. Here, I want to see if you can do it twice with the same weight. This will stimulate your muscular endurance fibers. They may be small, but don't forget them.

Exercise	Sets (11)	Reps
T-Bar Row	4	15, 15, 12, 6
Chins (to front)	4	To failure
Pulldown (to rear)	3	4, 20, 20

High Plains Deadlifter

If you haven't performed higher rep deadlifts (something beyond the typical 4-6 reps), you're in for an awakening. Higher reps doesn't necessarily mean you should use a relatively light weight. Use as much weight as possible. If you can get one more rep on these deadlifts sets, the weight isn't heavy enough. Just to make things even more challenging, I'll use the pullovers to pre-fatigue your lats before the deadlifts.

Exercise	Sets (14)	Reps
Dumbbell Pullover	3	12, 8, 6
Deadlift	3	12, 10, 8
Pulldown (neutral grip)	5	8, 8, 8, 8, 8
Pulldown (to rear)	3	10, 6, 10

Tree of Woe

Finish your back workout by hanging from a chinning bar for as long as you can. This is not a dead hang. Take a wide grip, contract your lats so you rise up a few inches and hold it there. Try it with and without lifting straps and note your hang time. After you fail and drop back to Earth, you might have a kinship with a flying tree squirrel.

Shoulders

The cornerstone of the deltoid workouts are presses of all types to give you the overall mass, while various lateral movements will provide more targeted mass building results. The key here is to almost always perform presses first in order to use maximum weights and to vary the order that the various lateral movements are performed in order to achieve symmetry and a stable shoulder structure.

Foundation I

Exercise	Sets (14)	Reps
Seated Dumbbell Press	5	15, 12, 10, 8, 6
Standing DB Front Raise	3	8-12
Standing DB Side Lateral	3	6-10
Rear Delt Machine	3	8-12

Foundation II

Exercise	Sets (14)	Reps
Standing Barbell Military Press	5	15, 12, 10, 8, 6
Standing Barbell Front Raise	3	8-12
Seated Dumbbell Side Lateral	3	8-12
Bent-over DB Rear Lateral	3	8-12

Devil in the Delts

This workout will be very quick. Only 10 sets, but the last six drop sets will leave you winded and your delts on fire. You may even hate the number six after this one. No front raises since the Military presses should be performed as heavy as possible (after warm-ups) which is plenty for your front delts.

Exercise	Sets (10)	Reps
Seated Barbell Military Press	4	6, 6, 6, 6
Standing DB Side Lateral	3	6>6>6, 6>6>6, 6>6>6
Standing Bent-over DB Lateral	3	6>6>6, 6>6>6, 6>6>6

Hold the Presses

This time we're going to pre-exhaust the front delts with front raises, then have you perform some very heavy Military presses standing. That will take everything you've got. The rear delts will get hit with an unusual exercise, standing Pulldown to the face—just concentrate on form and stability here and really squeeze those rear delts in the fully contracted position. You should feel an intense burn in the rear delts and see them pop out. Finally, a devilish ending to cap off the workout.

Exercise	Sets (13)	Reps
Barbell Front Raise	3	12, 12, 12
Standing BB Military Press	2	Warm ups
Standing BB Military Press	3	4, 4, 4
Standing Pulldown (to face)	3	15, 15, 15
Standing DB Side Lateral	2	6>6>6, 6>6>6

Bring up the Rear

This is a great workout to bring up lagging rear delt development, simply by starting with a rear delt movement. Give it everything you have. Next, you get to sit down and use the guidance of the Smith Machine—but notice you'll go really heavy here and hit the entire spectrum of rep ranges. The side laterals can be performed two ways—either really strict or with a little cheating momentum. If cheating, then use more weight than you could strictly. Finally, apply a brutal lift at the end-again, either strict or cheating—your choice.

Exercise	Sets (16)	Reps
Rear Delt Machine	4	15, 12, 10, 10
Smith Machine Military Press	6	15, 12, 10, 8, 6, 4
One-Arm DB Side Lateral	3	12, 10, 8
Barbell Front Raise	3	5, 5, 5

Traps

Shrugging movements build both your traps and your neck, while upright rows build the traps (and provide some good front delt, upper pec, and trap tie-ins). Therefore, the workouts presented here involve shrugs and upright rows performed with various apparatus and rep ranges in differing combinations.

Foundation I

Exercise	Sets (8)	Reps
Barbell or Dumbbell Shrug	4	6-15
Barbell Upright Row	4	8-12

Foundation II

Exercise	Sets (6)	Reps
Dumbbell Shrug	3	6
Barbell Shrug	3	8-10

Brutally Basic

You can't get more basic than this for traps. Pure barbell shrugs with heavy weight, extremely heavy weight, and a burn at the end. You will feel these tomorrow.

Exercise	Sets (8)	Reps
Barbell Shrug	8	8, 6, 3, 3, 6, 8, 15, 15

Reverse Attack

Performing shrugs and upright rows behind your back was a favorite of 8-time Mr. Olympia Lee Haney. Can't argue with those traps. Give these a try when you need something different or when your lower back is fatigued. Don't sacrifice form for weight on the upright rows. Make sure you can pull them as far up your back as possible.

Exercise	Sets (6)	Reps
Barbell Shrug (behind back)	3	6, 6, 6
Upright Row (behind back)	3	10, 10, 10

Upright Logic

To mix things up a bit, start with upright rows using a cable. That will give you more of a constant tension feel when doing these versus a bar. Then, off to the shrugs. Notice that the barbell shrugs are very, very heavy. Do them in a power rack.

Exercise	Sets (9)	Reps
Cable Upright Row	3	6-10
Barbell Shrug	3	4-6
Dumbbell Shrug	3	6-8

Ride the Rails

This is a great trap workout for a couple reasons. If you have a strain or muscle pull in your shoulder or upper back, the Smith Machine will keep you in a groove and in action and not on the sidelines. If all systems are go, then you can use very heavy weights and even some spotters to really overload the traps. Since some Smith Machines have a slight backward angle, this provides another variation, allowing you to pull up and slightly back. Tiny angular changes like this can sometimes make a big difference.

Exercise	Sets (6)	Reps
Smith Machine Shrug	6	15, 8, 8, 8, 8, 15

Biceps

Complete biceps workouts should try to include several things: an exercise with supination, a barbell curl of some sort, and brachialis/brachioradialus activation (reverse or hammer-type grips). The biceps workouts in this section should provide plenty of variety in these areas.

Foundation I

Exercise	Sets (9)	Reps
Standing Barbell Curl	3	6-8
Dumbbell Curl	3	8-12
Reverse Curl	3	6-12

Foundation II

Exercise	Sets (9)	Reps
Dumbbell Curl	3	6-8
Hammer Curl	3	6-8
Preacher Curl	3	10-12

Drop-Dead Arms

Not only do you have to contend with three early drop-sets in this workout, but also heavy weights and low reps throughout. Watch out for that last 10-rep set on the preacher curls—your struggle to maintain a decent weight there will be critical. Another final twist here is the low reps on the concentration curls, which is not typical.

Exercise	Sets (11)	Reps
Barbell Curl	5	10, 10, 6>6, 6>6, 6>6
Barbell Preacher Curl	3	5, 5, 10
DB Concentration Curl	3	6, 6, 6

Let's Hear it for the Barbell

An exclusive barbell workout for your biceps. Damn the supination, but they won't forget it.

Exercise	Sets (9)	Reps
Barbell Curl	3	6>6, 6>6, 6>6
Barbell Preacher Curl	3	6, 6, 6
Barbell Spider Curl	3	12, 10, 10

Unlucky

Nothing like starting with some barbell 21's, seven reps through each range of motion (bottom half, upper half, full range), to get you fired up. Then, sit down and don't relax through more partial rep curls. Finish up quickly with some peaking and brachialis work.

Exercise	Sets (9)	Reps
Barbell Curl 21's	2	21, 21
Barbell Curl (seated)	3	10, 10, 10
DB Concentration Curl	2	8, 8
Hammer Curl	2	8, 8

All Over the Place

This workout will have you standing, sitting, doing partial reps and crying by the end.

Exercise	Sets (13)	Reps
Barbell Curl	5	15, 10, 8, 6, 6
Hammer Curl	3	8, 8, 4
BB Preacher Curl (bottom half only)	3	12, 10, 8
Dumbbell Curl (seated)	2	6, 6

One-Arm Bandit

A typical start to this one, then it's all one-arm action with dumbbells and cables.

Exercise	Sets (12)	Reps
Barbell Curl	4	10, 10, 8, 4
One-Arm DB Preacher Curl	4	10, 10, 8, 6
One-Arm Cable Concentration Curl	4	10, 8, 6, 6

E-Z Does It

Every once in a while, it's good to take a break from standard barbell curls. While the E-Z bar won't get you that full supination as with a bar, the slight change in angle will get your attention.

Exercise	Sets (11)	Reps
E-Z Bar Curl	5	15, 12, 10, 6, 6
Barbell Preacher Curl	3	6, 6, 6
Hammer Curl	3	8, 6, 6

Zottman Lives!

The Zottman curl is an oft-neglected tool in the arsenal of bicep development. You get supination and a reverse curl in one movement—quite the bargain, especially if you're short on time. Oh, and if you haven't noticed, you've got a 20-rep set to finish out the preacher curls. That will definitely keep your biceps guessing.

Exercise	Sets (12)	Reps
Dumbbell Curl	5	12, 10, 6, 6, 8
Barbell Preacher Curl	3	5, 5, 20
DB Concentration Curl	2	6, 6
Zottman Curl	2	8, 8

Hang Tight

Reverse-grip chins performed with a close-grip are one of the most basic biceps builders around. Too bad next to no one does them. Here you change that and teach your fellow gym members a lesson. They'll also be staring when you do the lying dumbbell curls on a bench. That will give you a unique feel.

Exercise	Sets (11)	Reps
Reverse-Grip Chins (close grip)	3	To failure
Preacher Curl (EZ bar)	4	12, 12, 8, 8
Lying Dumbbell Curl	3	10, 10, 10
Incline Curl	1	15

At Arms Length

Nothing special here, except for the high rep preacher curls and your attempt to finish the bicep workout with close-grip chins—to failure.

Exercise	Sets (9)	Reps
Dumbbell Curl	3	12, 10, 8
Barbell Preacher Curl	3	15, 15, 15
Chins (close grip)	3	To failure

Great Scott

This is Larry Scott's famous biceps tri-set. It's brutal, so the first time you do this workout, just perform 3 tri-sets and work up from there. The key here is how you perform each exercise. Use maximum weights throughout. On the first exercise, place you elbows high up on the bench's pad and use any cheating necessary to get the six reps. Immediately pick up the barbell and sink your armpits into the top of the bench for the second exercise. This one you must do extremely strictly, especially the start of each rep. Absolutely no cheating here. Finally, pick up the E-Z bar and perform it just like the first exercise. If done correctly, this workout will provide you with an immense pump and some seriously soreness the next day.

Exercise	Sets (3-5 tri-sets)	Reps
Dumbbell Preacher Curl (loose)	3-5	6
Barbell Preacher Curl (strict)	3-5	6
Reverse E-Z Bar Curl (loose)	3-5	6

Ain't No Mountain High Enough

This one emphasizes biceps peak throughout. Start with relatively moderate weights on the cable crossover curls—you're just working to establish a pump here. The preacher curl will really hit the apex of your bicep, producing full, football-shaped development. Finally, nothing hits the peak like spider curls, especially since it's so hard to cheat with them.

Exercise	Sets (11)	Reps
Cable Crossover Curl	3	10-12
Barbell Preacher Curl	4	8-12
Spider Curls (BB or DB)	4	10-12

Peak Intensity

This workout emphasizes the development of your biceps peak using continuous tension cable exercises and the spider curl.

Exercise	Sets (14)	Reps
One-Arm Cable Curl	8	12, 12, 12, 12, 12, 10, 8, 4
Cable Crossover Curl	3	10, 8, 10
Dumbbell Spider Curl	3	10, 8, 8

Diversity Day

High reps, low reps, cable, dumbbell and barbell exercises. Standing and seated. A diverse workout to completely confuse your biceps into growth.

Exercise	Sets (12)	Reps
One-Arm Cable Curl	4	15, 12, 8, 4
Dumbbell Preacher Curl	2	6, 8
Barbell Curls (seated)	3	12, 10, 6
Barbell Spider Curl	3	6, 6, 6

Crazy Train

This workout must have been designed by a madman. Six different exercises, using some very high reps and a negative bombing run within. See if you can make it through. Some may be mad, but others just want to see your arms burn.

Exercise	Sets (15)	Reps
Preacher Curl (E-Z Bar)	1	30
BB Preacher Curl 21's	4	21, 21, 21, 21
BB Preacher Curl	1	3 negatives
Reverse Preacher Curl	3	12, 12, 12
E-Z Bar Curl	3	15, 12, 10
Seated DB Concentration Curl	3	8, 8, 8

Triceps

The most effective workouts for triceps typically involve close-grip presses, dips, extensions and pushdowns. You'll get that and a whole lot more in this section. Two things are critical to remember here—your triceps represent two-thirds of your total upper arm mass, and the long head of the triceps is the biggest of the triceps muscles. Keeping that in mind, work your triceps harder than your biceps and regularly involve an extension movement, which places your elbows above your head to pre-stretch the long head. Do this for a while, and everybody will wonder how your arms got so big. Time to get some new shirts.

Foundation I

Exercise	Sets (12)	Reps
Close-Grip Bench Press	4	12, 10, 8, 6
Lying or Standing Extension	4	6-12 reps
Pushdown	4	8-15 reps

Foundation II

Exercise	Sets (12)	Reps
Dips	4	8-12 reps (add weight if necessary)
Lying or Standing Extension	4	6-10 reps
Pushdowns	4	8-15 reps

Familiar Stranger

Familiarity can be a deceiving mistress. While this workout looks an awful lot like Foundation I, once you get going, a completely different feel emerges. A little more sets on the press, with peaks and valleys of reps, the feel of a heavy dumbbell in your hands for the extension, and the reappearance of a friend at the end.

Exercise	Sets (11)	Reps
Close-Grip Bench Press	5	15, 8, 6, 4, 20
Seated Dumbbell Extension	3	6, 6, 6
Pushdowns	3	12, 10, 8

For Good Measure(ment)

This workout has a little more volume than the Foundation workouts, since we throw two types of extension movements at you, in addition to the close-grip presses and pushdowns. For good measure, some higher reps are included this time around as well.

Exercise	Sets (14)	Reps
Close-Grip Bench Press	5	15, 12, 10, 6, 20
Lying E-Z Bar Extension	3	10, 8, 6
Dumbbell Extension (seated)	3	15, 15, 15
Pushdowns	3	8, 8, 8

The Final Countdown

Sometimes it's good to use the Smith Machine for your close-grip presses. Like when you want to go heavy but don't have a spotter—or you are managing a slight shoulder injury. A simple but effective triceps builder workout, with a final set that will scorch you.

Exercise	Sets (11)	Reps
Smith Close-Grip Bench Press	5	15, 15, 15, 6, 8
Pushdowns	6	12, 12, 12, 8, 8, 40

Extend Yourself

Just presses and extensions here, with a slight emphasis on the extensions. Notice that you'll perform the extensions both lying and seated, with a bar and dumbbells for added variety.

Exercise	Sets (11)	Reps
Smith Close-Grip Bench Press	5	12, 12, 12, 8, 6
Lying Extension (E-Z bar)	3	10, 8, 6
Dumbbell Extension (seated)	3	8, 8, 8

A Growing Sense of Doom

Very simple. Just do ten sets of twenty reps of extensions. The soreness will follow you for days like a beggar, and be etched in your memory long after he's gone.

Exercise	Sets (10)	Reps
Lying Extension (BB or E-Z bar)	10	10 sets of 20

Back to the Future

Before fancy equipment, like cable machines and E-Z bars appeared, muscular men of yore built massive triceps with the pullover and press, for good reason. It's a demanding exercise, which works the long head through an unusual angle, topped off with a close-grip pressing finish. I'll also throw in some high intensity drop-sets on the pushdowns and end with a futuristic cable extension. Bring back the memories and feel the hurt.

Exercise	Sets (12)	Reps
Barbell Pullover & Press	4	5, 5, 5, 5
Pushdowns	4 drop sets	[6 > 6] x 4 (one drop in weight per set)
Overhead Cable Extension	4	10, 8, 4, 4

Trifecta

There is nothing like tri-sets for the triceps for a muscular shock, especially one that uses high reps all the way around. Just use your body weight on the dips. You won't have enough time within the tri-set to strap on a dipping belt, and you probably won't need it by then either.

Exercise	Sets (5 tri-sets)	Reps
Pushdowns	5	15, 15, 15, 15, 15
Lying Barbell Extension	5	15, 15, 15, 15, 15
Dips	5	To failure

Max Pain

This is one tough mother. You've got high volume, some high reps, some low reps, drop-sets in an unusual position, while finishing with an exercise you usually start with. See how much basic pressing power you have left on that last six-rep set. It may be a humbling experience.

Exercise	Sets (15)	Reps
Decline Barbell Extension	4	15, 10, 6, 6
Pushdowns	4	10, 10, 10, 10
High Cable Extensions (kneeling)	4	15>15, 15>15, 10>10, 6>6
Close-Grip Bench Press	3	10, 8, 6

High Low

This workout starts with a high rep set to get you warmed up and ends with a high rep set to complete the final burn. In between are lots of very heavy, low-rep sets to build the muscle.

Exercise	Sets (15)	Reps
Pushdown (rope)	3	25, 10, 10
Lying E-Z Bar Extension	4	6, 6, 6, 6
Incline E-Z Bar Extension	3	6, 6, 6
Close-Grip Bench Press	4	6, 6, 6, 6
Pushdowns	1	30

No Loitering

You won't be standing around during this workout. Instead, you'll be cruising through some lengthy high-rep sets across four different exercises. The pump you achieve with the higher reps will assist you when pressing the crushing weight you need to use on the close-grip presses.

Exercise	Sets (12)	Reps
Seated One-Arm DB Extension	3	25, 20, 15
Lying E-Z Bar Extension	3	15, 12, 8
Close-Grip Bench Press	4	4, 4, 4, 20
Dips	2	To failure

Boomerang

You'll start and end this workout with a set of 20 rep pushdowns. Slightly higher reps all around make this a good workout if your elbows or shoulders need a break.

Exercise	Sets (10)	Reps
Pushdowns	4	20, 15, 12, 10
Lying Barbell Extension	5	15, 12, 10, 8, 6
Pushdowns	1	20

Alter Ego

This is a very typical triceps workout with a few key alterations. First, I want you to perform the extensions seated with a barbell—don't reach for the E-Z bar here. On the dips, strap on the dipping belt, because you need to go really heavy. If you can get seven reps, there's not enough weight on the belt.

Exercise	Sets (11)	Reps
Pushdowns	5	12, 12, 12, 6, 6
Seated Barbell Extensions	2	12, 12
Dips	4	6, 6, 6, 6

Reach for the Sky

Here we have the same type of exercises as Alter Ego, except you'll switch the order of the dips and extensions and replace the barbell with a dumbbell. You can stand for the extensions if you want to use a little cheating at the end, or sit and do them strictly all the way through.

Exercise	Sets (11)	Reps
Pushdowns	3	15, 12, 8
Dips	3	6, 6, 6
One-Arm Dumbbell Extension	5	8, 8, 8, 8, 8

Stand, Lie and Deliver

This workout features a combination exercise of extensions, immediately followed by presses. Just make sure you are close to failure on both before you stop.

Exercise	Sets (10)	Reps
Pushdowns	4	15, 12, 10, 8
Lying E-Z Bar Extension/Press	3	12/12, 6/6, 6/6
Seated Dumbbell Extension	3	8, 8, 8

Quick and the Dead

If you're short on time and big on pain, this workout is for you. Only eight sets with mainly low reps. Since you've only got one shot on that last exercise, make it count.

Exercise	Sets (8)	Reps
Seated Dumbbell Extension	4	6, 6, 6, 12
Close-Grip Bench Press	3	5, 5, 5
Lying E-Z Bar Extension	1	10

Forearms

Generally, if you don't use lifting straps, you'll find that you probably don't need any direct forearm work. Holding onto heavy barbells and dumbbells tends to develop the forearms along the journey. However, if you were genetically cheated in this area or you do use lifting straps consistently, then here are some effective workouts you can use to bring up this area.

Foundation I

Exercise	Sets (8)	Reps
Barbell Wrist Curls	4	6-15
Barbell Reverse Wrist Curls	4	6-15

Foundation II

Exercise	Sets (8)	Reps
Dumbbell Wrist Curls	4	6-15
Barbell Reverse Curls	4	6-8

Forearms of the Forefathers

Weightlifters of the 1940s and 1950s sported some impressively big and strong forearms—again, due mainly to the lack of lifting straps, and lots of heavy deadlifts and shrugs. They also typically included direct forearm work all of the time—remember, many of these lifters also performed feats of strength for beachside audiences. Strong forearms were a requirement. Barbells were the favored tool of choice and the barbell reverse curl, performed heavy helped them build massive and functional forearms that could lift objects and people from any angle. Every so often, perform the reverse curls with as much weight as possible, with slightly looser, cheating form for an additional overload.

Exercise	Sets (8)	Reps
Barbell Wrist Curls	4	6-8
Barbell Reverse Curls	4	6-8

Hold My Pencil

Perform these two exercises as a superset. What you are looking for here is a pump and burn in your forearms so great, that at the end of the four supersets you should have trouble with your fine motor skills.

Exercise	Sets (4 supersets)	Reps
Behind Back Wrist Curls	4	10
Reverse Curls	4	10

Divide and Conquer

It's typical for one forearm (your dominant arm) to be slightly larger and stronger than the other. This workout uses dumbbells to help you correct that asymmetry and provides a nice, higher rep pump. It's also about the most volume you should need for a forearm workout.

Exercise	Sets (10)	Reps
Dumbbell Reverse Wrist Curls	5	10-15
Dumbbell Wrist Curls	5	10-15

Grip of Steel

This is about as simple as it gets. Grab the heaviest dumbbells you can grip (without straps) or load up a barbell with more weight than you can shrug and hold on as long as your grip holds out. This is a great finisher to any type of upper body workout. If you've relied on straps for most of your lifting career, this is a good method to wean yourself off and build up that innate gripping power that lies within. Just try not to crush the hands of mere mortals that you interact with on a daily basis.

Exercise	Sets (3)	Reps
Barbell or Dumbbells	3	Hold onto the barbell or dumbbells as long as you can

Walk About

This workout is similar to Grip of Steel, except now you are going to walk around your gym until your grip gives out. Make sure you control the drop of the dumbbells onto a rubberized floor—you don't want to lose your toes or your membership.

Exercise	Sets (3)	Reps
Dumbells	3	Walk around the gym as long as your grip holds out

Quads

You can build massive, muscular, shapely and symmetrical quads with relatively few exercises. In fact, traditional squats alone have built many outstanding legs. The most result-producing quad workouts are based around leg extensions to warm the knee joints and provide pre-fatigue, and various squat and leg press movements. That's it. What is surprising is the number of effective workout permutations you can derive from those few, simple movements. Here they are.

Foundation I

Exercise	Sets (16)	Reps
Leg Extensions	4	6-15
Squats	4	4-15
Front Squats	4	6-12
Leg Press	4	6-15

Foundation II

Exercise	Sets (15)	Reps
Leg Press	3	10-20
Squats	5	6-12
Hack Squats	4	8-12
Leg Extension	3	6-12

Changes: Part I

You are only as strong in the squat as your weakest stance. This workout challenges you with your standard width squats at very heavy weights, followed by more squats with your stance both wide and narrow. Consistent use of this methodology will eliminate any stance weaknesses you may have.

Exercise	Sets (13)	Reps
Leg Extension	3	12, 10, 8
Squat	4	10, 8, 4, 2
Squat (narrow stance)	3	10
Squat (wide stance)	3	10

Changes: Part II

Here we continue with the motif of varying squat stance widths and throw in some heavy leg presses at the end.

Exercise	Sets (14)	Reps
Leg Extension	3	12, 10, 8
Squat	4	12, 6, 6, 10
Squat (narrow stance)	2	10
Squat (wide stance)	2	10
Leg Press	3	6

Do You Feel Lucky?

Although this may appear to be a low-volume workout that you can complete relatively quickly, you'll find out that may not be the case when you hit the six sets of 10 you need to do in the squat. That will tax you, but the coup de grace is the final set of Squat 21's. You can perform either the top or bottom half of the movement for the first seven reps, but always be sure to perform the full range squat for the final seven reps.

Exercise	Sets (10)	Reps
Leg Extension	3	10, 8, 6
Squat	6	10, 10, 10, 10, 10, 10
Squat 21's	1	21

Double Impact

Squats are demanding. Supersets with squats are borderline crazy. Here, you'll use a very heavy weight for partials squats, followed immediately by moderate weight full range squats. Repeat five times. Try to set up two separate squat racks with the different weights so you can immediately go from one to the other. Otherwise, you'll need to quickly change the weight each time, which will decrease the effectiveness of this workout.

Exercise	Sets (10)	Reps
Leg Extension	5	15, 12, 10, 8, 6
Squat (partials) / Squats	5	8 reps on the partials followed by 8 full range reps

Bottom's Up

Most lifters don't go to parallel when they squat. Almost none go below parallel. Subsequently, they develop weak adductors and limited flexibility, which ultimately limits the amount of weight they can handle with full range squats and doesn't allow them to reach their genetic potential of quad mass. This workout aims to correct that. You're going to spend a lot of time in the bottom portion of the squat movement here. For each rep, squat down to below parallel and come up only halfway to a full range squat. Learn to love the bottom—and don't cheat yourself.

Exercise	Sets (13)	Reps
Leg Extension	5	15, 12, 10, 8, 6
Squat	5	8 reps at bottom half of movement
Leg Press	3	10

Coronation

There are times in your workout career when you elevate yourself to new standards. This is one of those opportunities. Ascend to your throne.

Exercise	Sets (15)	Reps
Leg Extension	5	15, 12, 10, 8, 6
Squat	10	10, 10, 10, 10, 10, 10, 10, 10, 10, 10

The End of Insanity

Insanity is often manifested by abnormal behavior. In this case, I want you to go insane on the last set of this workout. You may need to roll off the leg press into the fetal position and eventually crawl back into the locker room after it's over. Needless to say, use as much weight as possible on that last set.

Exercise	Sets (12)	Reps
Leg Extension	4	15, 12, 10, 8
Squat	4	12, 10, 8, 6
Front Squat	3	10, 8, 6
Leg Press	1	100

The Outer Limits

One of the differentiating features between good quads and great quads is the amount of outer sweep in the quads. It's true that genetics play a large role in this area—however, I've found that most lifters just don't know how to maximize their potential here. The key to outer sweep is consistent use of front and hack squats—the two best exercises for developing the quad sweep. Since most people don't like to do front squats—well, you get good quads, but not great. For the hack and front squats in this workout, alternate your stance from wide to narrow from set to set.

Exercise	Sets (15)	Reps
Leg Extensions (narrow)	5	6-15
Hack Squats (wide/narrow)	5	6-12
Front Squats (wide/narrow)	5	6-12

Don't Cry for Me Medialis

The counterpart to great quad sweep is having a well-defined teardrop on the inner quad. This workout will really build up the teardrop (that's the vastus medialis, for you anatomy geeks out there).

Exercise	Sets (14)	Reps
Leg Extension (wide)	4	15, 12, 10, 8
Squat (wide stance)	3	10-12
Lunges	4	6-10
Front Squats (wide stance)	3	8-10

World's Apart

The only easy part to this workout is the first (and only) set of leg extension, just to get your knees warmed up. From there, it's just squats with varied stances, and partial range leg presses. On each rep, think of pushing the floor or Earth away from you. It's a good visualization to practice. You get lots of practice here.

Exercise	Sets (12)	Reps
Leg Extension	1	15
Squat	4	20, 15, 10, 5
Squat (narrow stance)	1	10
Squat (wide stance)	3	6 , 6, 6
Leg Press (bottom 3/4)	3	10, 10, 10

Foot Fetish

We've talked about the importance of changing foot stance widths when performing leg exercises. With this workout you'll place your feet wide, narrow, and normal widths apart. Also, be sure to use a weight on the leg press that you can't perform for full range reps. This will provide additional overload and growth.

Exercise	Sets (12)	Reps
Leg Extension	4	15, 12, 10, 6
Squat (wide stance)	4	12, 12, 6, 3
Leg Press (1/2 reps)	2	10, 10
Leg Press (feet close)	2	8, 8

Simpleton

Sometimes you don't feel like thinking. If it's leg day and that's how you feel, do this workout. Just leg extensions and standard squats with decreasing reps and increasing weight. Doesn't get much more basic and simple than that.

Exercise	Sets (11)	Reps
Leg Extension	3	15, 10, 8
Squat (wide stance)	8	15, 12, 6, 6, 6, 6, 6, 10

Simpleton's Cousin

Just like Simpleton, this one is a no brainer. You don't have to think about it, just do it.

Exercise	Sets (13)	Reps
Leg Extension	3	15, 12, 10
Front Squat (narrow/wide)	10	10 sets of 10

Press On

Here's our German Volume Training plan centered around the leg press this time. Each time you do this workout, try to increase the weight, even if by just ten pounds. Over time, those ten pounds add up. If you look down, you'll see the payoff.

Exercise	Sets (15)	Reps
Leg Extension	5	15, 15, 15, 10, 8
Leg Press	10	10 sets of 10

Endless

Looks like a typical volume-based 10 sets of 10 workout on the leg press. But, what makes this one different is the final exercise of Smith Machine squats with a narrow stance. You should feel the sides of your quads popping out when you do those sets.

Exercise	Sets (16)	Reps
Leg Extension	3	12, 12, 6
Leg Press	10	10 sets of 10
Smith Squat (narrow stance)	3	10, 10, 10

Palindrome

Here's a high-rep workout that's easy to remember, since it's a palindrome (the rep numbers are the same if the workout is reversed). It's also 200 reps of intensity.

Exercise	Sets (16)	Reps
Leg Extension	4	15, 15, 15, 15
Squat	4	10, 10, 10, 10
Hack Squat	4	10, 10, 10, 10
Angled Leg Press	4	15, 15, 15, 15

Finish What You Started

As usual, you'll save your knees by starting with leg extensions—but this workout also ends with leg extensions, performed one leg at a time for increased intensity.

Exercise	Sets (19)	Reps
Leg Extension	3	15, 12, 10
Squat	6	10, 10, 8, 6, 5, 5
Leg Press	4	12, 12, 12, 12
Hack Squat	3	8, 6, 6
Leg Extension (one leg)	3	10, 10, 10

Pump Up the Volume: Quad Edition

Here it is—the highest volume quad workout in this section. Try to reduce the time it takes you to complete the workout each time you make it through.

Exercise	Sets (23)	Reps
Leg Extension	4	15, 12, 8, 6
Hack Squat	5	10, 10, 6, 6, 6
Leg Press	7	10, 10, 10, 10, 8, 6, 6
Squat	5	6, 6, 6, 6, 6
Front Squat	2	5, 5

Pump Up the Volume: Quad Remix

Simply more high-volume goodness with plenty of variety for all tastes.

Exercise	Sets (21)	Reps
Leg Extension	4	20, 15, 8, 5
Squat	6	20, 12, 6, 6, 6, 6
Front Squat (wide stance)	4	10, 8, 6, 4
Angled Leg Press	4	10, 8, 6, 6
Hack Squat	3	8, 6, 6

Squataholic

You'll get an overdose of the most popular types of squat movements here. Just be glad we didn't throw in Jefferson or Zercher squats.

Exercise	Sets (17)	Reps
Leg Extension	4	15, 12, 10, 8
Squat (narrow stance)	5	15, 15, 12, 8, 6
Front Squat (wide stance)	5	8, 6, 4, 4, 4
Hack Squat (narrow stance)	3	10, 8, 6

WTF?

When we talk about performing a variety of rep ranges to hit all muscle fiber types, this is the type of workout we envision. You will go from the depths of a 4-rep set all the way to the excruciating muscular fatigue of a 30-rep set. Sort of like living a year in Springfield, Missouri (hint: Wikipedia).

Exercise	Sets (18)	Reps
Leg Extension	4	15, 12, 10, 8
Squat	7	20, 15, 12, 10, 8, 6, 30
Angled Leg Press	4	15, 12, 10,8
Front Squat	3	8, 6, 4

Dead Quads Walking

The first ten sets of this 11 set workout will get your quads pretty well fatigued. All you have left is to grab some heavy dumbbells and walk as far across the gym and back as you can. Try not to fall over.

Exercise	Sets (11)	Reps
Leg Extension	3	20, 15, 12
Smith Machine Squat	4	10, 8, 8, 8
Angled Leg Press	3	12, 10, 8
Dumbbell Lunge	1	Across the gym and back

Adventures in Squatting

Many people perform squats in their workouts. Fewer perform front squats. Even fewer have tried front squats on a Smith Machine. It provides a good break for those without spotters who still want to go heavy.

Exercise	Sets (14)	Reps
Leg Extension	3	20, 15, 10
Squat	5	10, 10, 10, 10, 10
Hack Squat	3	15, 5, 5
Smith Machine Front Squat	3	15, 5, 5

Super Squats Primer

Nothing puts on quad mass like sets of 20 rep squats—if you can survive. Just ask Randall Strossen, author of the seminal *Super Squats* book, first published in 1989.

Exercise	Sets (11)	Reps
Leg Extension	3	20, 12, 10
Squat (wide stance)	5	10, 10, 10, 10, 10
Front Squat	2	6, 6
Squat	1	20

High-Rep Wonder

Some individuals' quads respond better to higher reps. If that's you or you aren't sure if that is you, then try this one. You won't go below ten reps per set in this workout.

Exercise	Sets (12)	Reps
Leg Extension	5	15, 12, 10, 10, 10
Hack Squat	5	12, 12, 12, 10, 10
Squat	2	12, 12

iMachine

Sometimes you need a mental or physical break from putting that squat bar on your back or across your clavicles. If that's the case, then this all-machine quad workout will provide a tough, but guided respite.

Exercise	Sets (15)	Reps
Leg Extension	3	15, 15, 15
Hack Squat	3	12, 10, 10
Smith Machine Squat	3	8, 8, 8
Smith Machine Front Squat	3	6, 6, 6
Leg Press	3	8, 8, 8

True Grit

Front squats are tough enough to perform, from both performance and breathing aspects. Placing them last in your workout with heavy weights amplifies the intensity and further challenges your character. Do you have what it takes?

Exercise	Sets (16)	Reps
Leg Extension	4	15, 15, 15, 15
Hack Squat	4	10, 10, 3, 10
Smith Machine Squat	4	10, 5, 5, 5
Front Squat	4	6, 6, 6, 6

Weary Warrior

How about ten sets to pre-fatigue your quads before you get to the squat? I would highly recommend spotters for those sets of three reps by that point. They may need to carry you off the battlefield.

Exercise	Sets (15)	Reps
Leg Extension	5	15, 12, 12, 10, 8
Leg Press	5	20, 12, 12, 8, 6
Squat	5	10, 3, 3, 3, 10

Fear Factor

Often, what holds back your progress is your mind. This workout will test the strength of both your head and your heart. First, you have to set in your mind that you can do this—then, when your mind starts to doubt, let your heart take over. For the leg extensions you need to increase the weight each set AND increase the reps. For the squats, perform decreasing reps and increasing weight until you get to the first set of 12 reps. Pick a weight you think you can do for 10 reps and use that. Then, keep using that weight for the final two sets, including the 20-rep set. Confront your fears and grow.

Exercise	Sets (13)	Reps
Leg Extension	4	10, 12, 14, 16
Squat	9	15, 12, 4, 4, 4, 4, 12, 12, 20

Demolition Man

This is nine sets of pure grit and pain. Two exercises. The first two sets of squats should be a warm-up—those that follow should not. Load up the leg press as heavy as possible—will your head or heart pick that weight?

Exercise	Sets (9)	Reps
Squat	8	8, 6, 4, 4, 4, 4, 4, 4
Leg Press	1	30

I Am Number Five

Performing sets of five reps will condition your body for muscular power and pure strength. This is your modified power program centered on the front and hack squats with the gift of life at the end.

Exercise	Sets (15)	Reps
Squat	5	15, 15, 15, 10, 5
Front Squat	5	15, 5, 5, 5, 5
Hack Squat	5	5, 5, 5, 5, 20

Carry On

Sometimes the weak link in a squat workout arrives with lower back fatigue. If that is you, and today you are motivated, then performing supersets with barbell squats followed by Smith Machine squats will push you further without pushing your lower back over the edge.

Exercise	Sets (10)	Reps
Squat + Smith Machine Squat	6	15, 10, 10, 8, 6, 4
Leg Extension (one leg)	4	8, 8, 6, 6

Heavy Metal

This workout gets heavy real quick and stays heavy. A pure mass builder—even on the extensions.

Exercise	Sets (14)	Reps
Squat	8	15, 12, 3, 3, 3, 5, 5, 10
Front Squat	2	8, 6
Leg Extension	4	6, 6, 6, 6

Halfway There

Start with a warm-up set of 25 reps on the leg press. Then, perform a typical half-pyramid of squats. Now, what makes this workout different is the use of half-squats next—use a weight that you can't squat for a full range of motion. Be sure to keep your legs under continuous tension and not lock them out during each set of half-squats. After that deluge, switch to front squats and go all the way down and back up, adjusting the weight as necessary.

Exercise	Sets (12)	Reps
Leg Press	1	25
Squat	5	10, 8, 6, 6, 4
Squat (partial reps)	3	10, 10, 10
Front Squat (narrow stance)	3	3, 5, 12

Devilish

This is a high-volume workout where you'll spend about half your time performing heavy sets of squats and front squats with six reps. Also, you'll begin and end the workout with high-rep leg presses. Try to use a heavier weight for the final 25 reps than you used for the initial set.

Exercise	Sets (21)	Reps
Leg Press	1	25
Leg Extension	6	15, 15, 15, 8, 8, 8
Smith Machine Squat	8	6, 6, 6, 6, 6, 6, 6, 6
Front Squat	2	6, 6
Leg Press	4	15, 15, 15, 25

Confusability

In the end, sometimes you really need to change things up, confuse the muscles by doing everything different from the norm. This workout amps the volume, moves the rep range around, and changes the typical ordering of the exercises. You can change it further from here.

Exercise	Sets (18)	Reps
Leg Press	7	15, 12, 10, 8, 8, 8, 8
Squat	4	6, 6, 6, 6
Smith Machine Front Squat	3	20, 3, 3
Leg Extension	4	10, 10, 10, 10

Step Up

This is one of those rare workouts where you can actually use a cardio machine to build your glutes. If your gym has a Step Mill machine, then this will work great. Otherwise, you can improvise by using any other type of step machine or the treadmill on a high incline at low speed. In all cases, squeeze your glute hard on each step and exaggerate your range of motion—lift your leg high and then squeeze on the step. You can do this for five minutes at the end of each workout.

Exercise	Sets (9)	Reps
Step Ups (dumbbell)	4	10-15
Reverse Lunges	4	10-15
Step Machine	1	5 minutes

Hamstrings

Hamstring workouts are built around concentric contraction-based exercises (some type of leg curl) and eccentric extension/stretching exercises (a form of deadlifts, such as Romanian or Stiff-Leg). Most gyms only have one type of leg curl apparatus (typically a lying leg curl machine)—if you have more, consider yourself lucky. Old school weightlifters will remember the days of iron boots to perform their leg curls, which is one reason why hamstring development lagged relative to other body parts 40 or 50 years ago. Today, based on the limited variety of leg curl machines, you need to make adjustments in intensity, volume, and rep ranges to bust through any hamstring plateaus you may encounter. The tenaciously smart and clever hamstring technician will prevail here.

Foundation I

Exercise	Sets (8)	Reps
Lying Leg Curl	4	15, 12, 10, 8
Stiff-Leg Deadlift	4	6-12

Foundation II

Exercise	Sets (10)	Reps
Stiff- Leg Deadlift	5	6-12
Lying Leg Curl	5	6-12

Opposite Realms

Same exercises as Foundation I, but changes in the rep range make a world of difference. The opening set of 30 reps on the curls will sufficiently warm your hamstrings for the heavy siege you need to lay on them for the following three sets. You'll finish by stretching things out a bit.

Exercise	Sets (7)	Reps
Lying Leg Curl	4	30, 5, 5, 5
Stiff-Leg Deadlift	3	10, 10, 10

Old Reliable

This is a workout I come back to quite often. It never fails to produce results. It just has the right amount of volume and rep ranges.

Exercise	Sets (10)	Reps
Lying Leg Curl	6	8, 8, 4, 6, 6, 20
Stiff-Leg Deadlift	4	12, 6, 6, 6

Concentration

If you've never performed concentration leg curls on the lying machine, here's how to do it. Lie down on the machine as you normally would. Then, extend your arms so they are straight—your upper body should now be off the pad, while your hips and thighs remain in contact. Keeping this rigid position, curl the weight up and hold the contraction for a second or two. Think of this as spider curls for the hamstrings. You'll end up with the same effect. You'll also notice that you can't use anywhere near the amount of weight you would normally do. This is ok. Just concentrate on form and contraction.

Exercise	Sets (7)	Reps
Lying Concentration Leg Curl	4	6-10
Stiff-Leg Deadlift	3	6-8

Improvisation

Here we introduce the standing leg curl into the workout. If your gym doesn't have a standing leg curl machine, you can improvise by using the leg extension machine by standing and facing the machine's seat with your thigh against the edge of the seat. Place your calf against the extension pad and curl the extension arm upwards.

Exercise	Sets (8)	Reps
Standing Leg Curl	4	15, 6, 6, 6
Stiff-Leg Deadlift	4	12, 12, 12, 12

Sir Mix a Lot

Now that you know how to improvise with standing leg curls if your gym doesn't have that apparatus, let's combine three different hamstring exercise in this workout.

Exercise	Sets (10)	Reps
Lying Leg Curl	5	12, 10, 6, 4, 6
Standing Leg Curl	2	8, 8
Stiff-Leg Deadlift	3	6, 6, 6

Heavy Hams

Lots of volume and heavy weights/low reps characterize this workout. Just for fun, I'll throw in a couple high rep sets to see if you can make it through.

Exercise	Sets (12)	Reps
Lying Leg Curl	7	6, 6, 6, 6, 6, 12, 25
Stiff-Leg Deadlift	5	6, 6, 6, 6, 6

Stand By Me

Now we add in more volume and a really heavy set to the standing leg curl. You'll also get an immediate pump and burn from the first set of lying leg curls, which may make it a tough go on the following four sets. Stay with it.

Exercise	Sets (11)	Reps
Lying Leg Curl	5	30, 10, 10, 10, 10
Standing Leg Curl	6	12, 10, 8, 4, 15, 15

Quick Fire Challenge

If you are short on time to work your hamstrings, this workout will produce effective results. The 20-rep set is what makes the last two sets a challenge. Are you up to it? This is also a nice workout to do after your quad workout, especially if you are doing supplemental hamstring work, in addition to your regular ham workout, to bring them up.

Exercise	Sets (6)	Reps
Standing Leg Curl	4	8, 6, 6, 20
Lying Leg Curl	2	6, 8

May I Have Three?

This workout is similar to the Foundation workouts, except for two things—the opening high-rep set and the extremely heavy set of three reps, after your hams are warm. Use as much weight as you possibly can here. It's good every once in a while to shock the hams with a very low rep set like this. They can take it.

Exercise	Sets (7)	Reps
Lying Leg Curl	4	20, 15, 3, 10
Stiff-Leg Deadlift	3	8, 8, 8

Engorged

The high reps in this workout will keep the blood pumping into your hams. By the final set, you'll have about as much blood in them as they can take.

Exercise	Sets (7)	Reps
Lying Leg Curl	4	15, 12, 10, 8
Stiff-Leg Deadlift	3	15, 15, 15

20 Rep Hamstrings

Short and intense. Nothing better describes this workout. Once you master your three sets of 20, try increasing the weight each time you do this workout, or try to reduce your rest intervals.

Exercise	Sets (3)	Reps
Stiff-Leg Deadlift	3	20, 20, 20

Pump Up the Volume: Hamstring Edition

You've seen variations of this one many times before. We're going for high volume here. The lying leg curls will provide your heavy low-rep training. Everything else will feel like pure fire.

Exercise	Sets (15)	Reps
Seated Leg Curl	5	15, 15, 15, 10, 5
Lying Leg Curl	5	8, 6, 6, 6, 6
Stiff-Leg Deadlift	5	10, 10, 10, 10, 10

Two Sacks of Concrete

Most of the time, you'll do your stiff-leg deadlifts with a barbell, since that is most effective for building mass and handling really heavy weights. Here, I'll switch things up a bit by using dumbbells. You can choose to hold the dumbbells in front of you or to the sides—if your lower back is sore, you should probably try the side option.

Exercise	Sets (9)	Reps
Lying Leg Curl	5	15, 15, 10, 10, 10
Dumbbell Stiff-Leg Deadlift	3	10, 6, 6

Two Sacks of Sand

Which is heavier, concrete or sand? Although similar to the workout above, you'll find that sand is a bit easier to take, since the dumbbell stiff-leg deadlifts are done first, when your energy is fresh, the reps are a bit higher and the weight should be a bit lighter.

Exercise	Sets (8)	Reps
Dumbbell Stiff-Leg Deadlift	4	12, 10, 10, 10
Standing Leg Curl	4	8, 4, 15, 12

10 Sets of 10

The name of the workout says it all. German Volume Training for the hams.

Exercise	Sets (10)	Reps
Lying Leg Curl	10	10, 10, 10, 10, 10, 10, 10, 10, 10, 10

Make It End

All you are going to do here is lying leg curls. The difference maker here will be the two sets of 20 reps at the end.

Exercise	Sets (8)	Reps
Lying Leg Curl	8	15, 12, 10, 8, 6, 6, 20, 20

Half Pyramid Hell

Nine sets of increasing weight and decreasing reps make this half pyramid something that you won't soon forget.

Exercise	Sets (9)	Reps
Lying Leg Curl	9	15, 12, 10, 8, 6, 4, 4, 6, 6

Negative Vibes

This is a simple, exclusive lying leg curl workout—until you get to the last two sets. Yes, you read that right—that's eight negative reps on each of the last two sets. You'll need someone to assist you with raising the curl pad as those sets progress, and to help you stand upright afterwards. Have a nice day.

Exercise	Sets (8)	Reps
Lying Leg Curl	8	15, 15, 10, 8, 6, 12, 8 negatives, 8 negatives

Helping Hams

Sometimes you just don't feel like doing stiff-leg deadlifts. Maybe your lower back is slightly sore, your oblique has a slight pull, or you just don't have the motivation. This is the time to rely on your friend, the Smith Machine. He will balance the bar and keep you locked into the same motion, so your lower back, obliques and psyche can have a respite. Just for good measure, let's keep the weight and reps moderate.

Exercise	Sets (9)	Reps
Smith Stiff-Leg Deadlift	5	10, 10, 10, 10, 10
Seated Leg Curl	2	8, 8
Lying Leg Curl	2	8, 8

Helping Hams II

A little less volume and fewer exercises than the original. But still tasty.

Exercise	Sets (8)	Reps
Smith Stiff-Leg Deadlift	4	12, 10, 8, 8
Lying Leg Curl	4	6, 6, 6, 6

Catching Up

One way to increase intensity on leg curls is to perform them one leg at a time. This also lets you test the relative strength of your hamstrings—one may be slightly stronger than the other. Now you know why that one is bigger, sort of like a stepbrother who lives with you. Use this knowledge and the intensity techniques in this book to unify the family into a symmetrical whole.

Exercise	Sets (8)	Reps
Lying Leg Curl (one leg)	4	15, 12, 10, 8
Stiff-Leg Deadlifts	4	15, 10, 6, 6

High Roller

Two things make this workout unique. The high rep range on the stiff-leg deadlifts and performing 21's for your hamstrings, a technique most often used with biceps. Wait a minute—hamstrings are like biceps. Hmm.

Exercise	Sets (7)	Reps
Stiff- Leg Deadlifts	4	15, 15, 15, 15
Lying Leg Curl 21's	3	21, 21, 21

Throne Room

This workout is humbling in two ways. The first half has you sitting and squeezing on your throne. You should be familiar with that by now. In the second portion, you will bow and rise up ten times, if you are worthy.

Exercise	Sets (8)	Reps
Seated Leg Curl	4	15, 10, 8, 8
Stiff-Leg Deadlift	4	10, 10, 10, 10

Super Stiff

This workout employs same exercise supersets, one with a barbell, and the other with a cable, to increase the intensity of your stiff-leg deadlifts. In essence, you'll be performing a combined 20 reps on each of those last three sets. Moving from the barbell to cable will provide continuous tension on those hams.

Exercise	Sets (8)	Reps
Lying Leg Curl	5	15, 12, 10, 8, 6
Stiff-Leg Deadlift / Cable Stiff-Leg Deadlift	3	10/10, 10/10, 10/10

May I Have Another?

If you can make it through the first two sets, you'll be close to the end of this workout. However, that tunnel at the end is a long, painful one.

Exercise	Sets (6)	Reps
Stiff-Leg Deadlift	2	25, 25
Lying Leg Curl	3	8, 8, 8
Seated Leg Curl	1	40

Rise Up

This workout is all about contracting your hamstrings to straighten your torso. While the stiff-leg deadlifts, performed with a moderate weight for sets of 12 reps will give you a good pump, the hamstring hyperextensions will provide a unique twist that will really tax you. Just use your body weight for the first set of hamstring hypers, then hold onto one or more plates to increase the effort so you can only get six reps. If you've never done these before, the key is to use only your hamstring contraction to pull you up—try not to contract your spinal erectors to lift yourself. It may take some practice, but you'll know you have it down when you feel soreness in your hamstrings and not your lower back then next day.

Exercise	Sets (8)	Reps
Stiff-Leg Deadlifts	4	12, 12, 12, 12
Hamstring Hyperextension	4	15, 6, 6, 6

Calves

There's not a whole lot of exercises for calves (roughly a half dozen or so) and most gyms typically only have two types of calf machines (seated and standing), therefore you really have to push the boundaries of intensity techniques, rep ranges, volume and creativity to achieve consistent muscle confusion in this area. This section will give you some ideas in this realm. I'll start with all the workouts that begin by primarily hitting the gastrocnemius, where your legs are almost locked out straight (this is where most of the variety of calf exercises lie), then move on to workouts that give priority to the diamond-shaped soleus, where you need to have your legs bent. The lack of exercise/machine diversity in that area will require some creativity. Oh, and there are lots of fire references in the workout titles for reasons that will become quite apparent.

Foundation I

Exercise	Sets (8)	Reps
Standing Calf Raise	4	6-20
Seated Calf Raise	4	6-20

Foundation II

Exercise	Sets (8)	Reps
Seated Calf Raise	4	10-20
Donkey Calf Raise	4	10-20

Long Fuse

This complete calf workout starts heavy and builds to a white-hot burn at the end.

Exercise	Sets (9)	Reps
Standing Calf Raise	4	6, 6, 6, 6
Seated Calf Raise	5	6, 10, 10, 25, 25

Roman Candle

While similar to Long Fuse, this workout flips the number of sets for these exercises, has slightly higher reps throughout and contains one final incendiary set that you must will yourself to get through.

Exercise	Sets (9)	Reps
Standing Calf Raise	5	12, 10, 8, 6, 6
Seated Calf Raise	4	12, 12, 12, 50

Gastro Delight I

This workout is all gastrocnemius, if you keep your legs almost straight. It's also a fairly heavy workout, and you'll probably need someone pretty heavy on your hips if you don't have access to a donkey calf raise machine.

Exercise	Sets (7)	Reps
Standing Calf Raise	4	12, 6, 6, 4
Donkey Calf Raise	3	8, 8, 8

Gastro Delight II

A similar serving to the workout above, except for one more set in volume, and a little bit more of the standing raise and a little less of the Donkeys. Throw in higher reps for the Donkeys and see how this one tastes.

Exercise	Sets (8)	Reps
Standing Calf Raise	6	8, 6, 6, 4, 4, 6
Donkey Calf Raise	2	15, 12

More Than Meets the Eye

Doesn't look like much, does it? How can just five sets do anything? The key here is the target number of reps, which equates to some really, really heavy weights. After properly warming up your calves, ankles, and Achilles tendon, and wrapping your mind around what you need to do, put that pin as far down the weight stack as you can and go to it. Don't sacrifice form for weight here and make sure to keep your body straight as an arrow.

Exercise	Sets (5)	Reps
Standing Calf Raise	5	6, 6, 6, 6, 6

Alternate Ending

A simple gastroc-only workout, with a high rep set at the end that makes the difference.

Exercise	Sets (7)	Reps
Standing Calf Raise	7	10, 6, 6, 6, 6, 8, 25

Flame Out

A quick gastroc-only workout, which starts with very high reps, giving you a quick pump and a white-hot burn. Try to increase the weights as much as possible through the rest of the sets.

Exercise	Sets (5)	Reps
Standing Calf Raise	5	40, 15, 12, 8, 8

Molotov Cocktail

This is a great calf workout if you are short on time. It's also a great workout you can use quickly at the start of any workout to bring up lagging calves. If you bend your legs a little, you can activate both the gastrocnemius and soleus effectively.

Exercise	Sets (3 drop)	Reps
Standing Calf Raise	3	10 > 10 > 10

Hold On

The key to this workout is getting 20 reps on all five sets with the same weight. Try to increase the weight you can use every week for best results.

Exercise	Sets (5)	Reps
Standing Calf Raise	5	20, 20, 20, 20, 20 (same weight on all sets)

Position is Everything

Every once in awhile we have to make even the most stubborn calves grow. This one will do it. The high rep opening set will prepare your calves for the monster weights you need for the remainder of your standing sets. After a quick respite on the seated calf raise, grab a hold of an upright from a machine, put your feet together and squat down until your hamstrings touch your calves. Using only your calves, rise up as high as you can to the balls of your feet and hold the contraction for a second. Come back to Earth and do it 24 more times.

Exercise	Sets (8)	Reps
Standing Calf Raise	5	30, 12, 5, 5, 5
Seated Calf Raise	2	15, 8
Squatting Calf Raise	1	25

Animalistic

In this workout you get to play the parts of a stork and a donkey, but don't feel like an ass while doing it. Performing calf raises one leg at a time while holding a dumbbell on the same side increases intensity and allows you to focus on any calf weakness.

Exercise	Sets (6)	Reps
Dumbbell One-Leg Calf Raise	3	12, 12, 12
Donkey Calf Raise	3	10, 10, 10

Angle of Attack

The 45° angled leg press is an effective calf builder, allowing you to work up to some very heavy poundages. This high-volume workout will start you on that exercise, building up the weight for the heavy sets of standing raises that follow. Finally, we can't forget the soleus, so after lying down and standing, you get to sit for the final three sets. Keep your legs as straight as possible on the calf press for the most effective results.

Exercise	Sets (13)	Reps
Angled Calf Press	5	25, 15, 6, 6, 3
Standing Calf Raise	5	5, 5, 5, 5, 5
Seated Calf Raise	3	15, 12, 10

Heavy Metal

The calf press will warm you up and pump you up for the heavy weight you need to handle to make this workout effective.

Exercise	Sets (8)	Reps
Angled Calf Press	4	35, 20, 15, 6
Standing Calf Raise	4	5, 5, 5, 5

Inflation

You'll lose nothing and have everything to gain in this quick single exercise calf workout. Loading and unloading the machine will take the most time here.

Exercise	Sets (6)	Reps
Angled Calf Press	6	15, 12, 8, 8, 8, 20

Pump Up the Volume: Calf Edition

You know the drill by now. At least double the number of sets you typically perform for calves. Works every time, as long as you don't do it every time.

Exercise	Sets (20)	Reps
Angled Calf Press	20	6-20

Supersize Me

Every once in awhile, you need to throw in some supersets for calves to give them the growth shock they need. Remember, calves aren't coaxed into growth, you have to force them with everything you've got. Low reps and supersets mean this workout will be over in no time—but the soreness will linger.

Exercise	Sets (5 Supersets)	Reps
Seated Calf Press	5	15, 8, 6, 6, 6
Standing Calf Raise	5	5, 5, 5, 5, 5

Old School

There's a reason why Arnold liked Donkey calf raises. They probably work better than any other exercise for building the gastrocnemius, since they really stretch the calves and allow you to get really high up on the balls of your feet. That's one serious range of motion. The only problem is finding appropriate and willing participants to sit on your hips. Arnold didn't have that problem—he often had three guys sitting on him. You'll be lucky to find one in this modern era.

Exercise	Sets (8)	Reps
Donkey Calf Raise	4	12, 6, 6, 12
Seated Calf Raise	4	12, 12, 20, 35

Solar Flare

This is the quickest workout for calves presented here. Just four sets, exclusively for the soleus. However, the intensity of the lactic acid burn will make you think you dipped your calves into the sun.

Exercise	Sets (4)	Reps
Seated Calf Raise	3	10, 10, 30
Squatting Calf Raise	1	25

Throne of Pain

Here's an entire workout dedicated to the soleus muscle. The descending rep range will provide you will ample time for your calves and mind to prepare for the five and three rep sets that will seal your fate. That's about as low as you ever want to go with reps for your calves, so make sure you only use this workout infrequently, lest your tendons betray you.

Exercise	Sets (8)	Reps
Seated Calf Raise	8	20, 15, 10, 8, 5, 3, 5, 8

5 Minute Calves

This is no infomercial. You'll need access to a watch or clock for this one. What you are going to do is note the start time (I like to wait until the second hand is at 12) and then start performing seated calf raises until you reach failure. Then rest 30 seconds and repeat. Every time you reach failure, check the time and rest 30 seconds. Keep doing this until five minutes have elapsed from your original start time. The key here is balancing the amount of weight you use, the number of reps you can average, and the number of sets you can perform in those five minutes. Play around with those variables and see what kind of results you get. Comes with a money-back guarantee that you will have a hard time walking immediately after finishing this one.

Exercise	Sets (?)	Reps
Seated Calf Raise	?	As many as you can do in 5 minutes

Recommended Reading

The following books contain a wealth of valuable information that was instrumental in developing the system described in this book (listed in order of recommendation):

- **The New Encyclopedia of Modern Bodybuilding** (Arnold Schwarzenneger and Bill Dobbins)

- **The Complete Keys to Progress** (John McCallum)

- **Loaded Guns** (Larry Scott)

- **The Strongest Shall Survive: Strength Training for Football** (Bill Starr)

- **Keys to the Inner Universe** (Bill Pearl)

Additionally, it may be very instructive and enlightening to research and read about the types of workouts and exercises used by bodybuilders and strongmen in the pre-1965 era—the time before anabolic steroids dominated weight lifting. I've included some of these workouts in each body part section above.

You'll find that men such as John Grimek, Steve Reeves, Reg Park, George Eiferman, and others, used fairly simple workouts based around compound, free weight movements to build incredibly dense muscularity and strength. What they didn't have at the time was access to low-fat, high protein supplementation sources, such as whey and casein protein powders and some of our more useful, modern pieces of exercise equipment, such as leg extensions and curls that are hard to duplicate with iron boots.

The Pearl and McCallum books above can get you started in this area.

Final Thoughts

If you thought this book was about weight training, you were wrong.

Supermen (and women!) are not defined by what they look like, but rather by their hearts and minds. Consistency, absolute effort, the ability to look at oneself honestly, and the continual thirst for new knowledge is what make them great.

You can be too.

The Supermen: 30 Years of Weight Training

Some of the current cadre, ranging in age from 23 to 54.

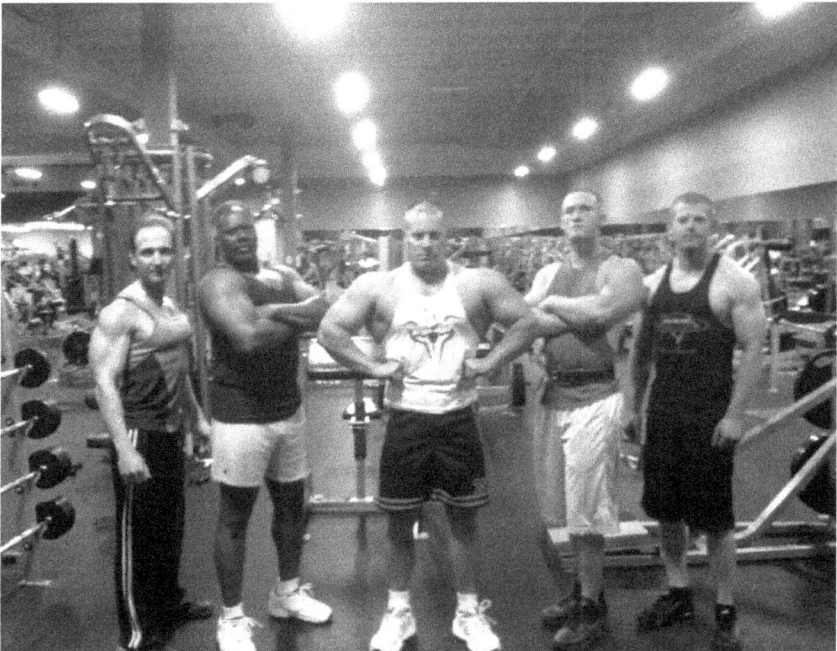

Pictured: Dave, Mitch, Craig, Adam and Kyle.

Additional Resources

Software for your Computer (PC or Mac)

If you liked this book, you may be interested in software, which supports the material you just read.

Running Deer Software (www.runningdeersoftware.com) provides low-cost spreadsheet and browser-based software for workout tracking and preparation, exercise selection, fitness testing, and diet analysis.

MuscleCALC

Weightlifting workout log and analysis system (spreadsheet).

FitnessCALC

Fitness assessment testing and tracking (spreadsheet).

Exercise Genie

Exercise encyclopedia and workout builder (spreadsheet).

Exercise Gambler

Random workout generation using a fun slot-machine game (browser app).

Diet Genie

Food database and nutritional analysis system (spreadsheet).

www.ingramcontent.com/pod-product-compliance
Lightning Source LLC
Chambersburg PA
CBHW062205270326
41930CB00009B/1655